Albanian
Escape

Albanian Escape

The True Story
of U.S. Army Nurses
Behind Enemy Lines

Agnes Jensen Mangerich

As Told to

Evelyn M. Monahan
and Rosemary L. Neidel

THE UNIVERSITY PRESS OF KENTUCKY

Publication of this volume was made possible in part by a grant from the National Endowment for the Humanities.

Published by The University Press of Kentucky

Scholarly publisher for the Commonwealth,
serving Bellarmine College, Berea College, Centre
College of Kentucky, Eastern Kentucky University,
The Filson Club Historical Society, Georgetown College,
Kentucky Historical Society, Kentucky State University,
Morehead State University, Murray State University,
Northern Kentucky University, Transylvania University,
University of Kentucky, University of Louisville,
and Western Kentucky University.
All rights reserved.

Editorial and Sales Offices: The University Press of Kentucky
663 South Limestone Street, Lexington, Kentucky 40508-4008

03 02 01 00 99   5 4 3 2 1

Library of Congress Cataloging-in-Publication Data

Mangerich, Agnes Jensen, 1914-
    Albanian escape : the true story of U.S. Army nurses behind
enemy lines / by Agnes Jensen Mangerich ; as told to
Evelyn M. Monahan and Rosemary L. Neidel.
        p.   cm.
    Includes bibliographical references.
    ISBN 0-8131-2109-4 (cloth : alk. paper)
    1. World War, 1939-1945—Medical care—United States.
2. Flight nursing—United States. 3. Nurses—United States—
History—20th century. 4. Escapes—Albania. I. Monahan, Evelyn.
II. Neidel, Rosemary L., 1941-   . III. Title.
D807.U6M357   1999
940.54'7573'092—dc21   98-48348

Written for my children,
Karen Anne and Jon Richard,
who would not be here today
without the many Albanians who helped
at peril of their own lives

Contents

Photographs follow page 130

Author's Note

Lost in bad weather, we crash-landed in German-occupied Albania, where we were hidden, led, and fed by Albanian partisans for sixty-two days. I carefully kept a diary on three tiny pieces of paper, logging as best I could names of towns, weather and walking conditions, and descriptions of those who helped us. This diary was taken away from me at our initial debriefing. It was later returned, and I added pages of details to flesh out my cryptic notes to insure that I would not forget about those who helped in our escape. Army Intelligence (G-2) told us that under no circumstances were we to talk freely about our ordeal or the escape procedures until they notified us and we were officially debriefed.

When I started to write about our ordeal in Albania, it was only to provide a complete framework to connect the snippets of information my children and friends had heard from me over the years. I wrote on legal tablets, filling several with recollections, and realized, maybe for the first time, what a raw struggle for survival it had been.

Although I wanted to provide a complete and accurate recounting, I wasn't interested in publication while the communist regime of Enver Hoxha was still in power in Albania. There were so many Albanians who had helped us in such a specific geographic area, and I did not want any repercussions for those who might be identified. In the late 1940s, Kostig Steffa, one of our English-speaking guides, had in fact been executed for his wartime activities. When the dictator Hoxha died in 1985, Albania slowly began to move toward democratic freedoms, and I began to think about publication as a reality.

Help came from my friend, Ruth Sowash, who was determined the story be told and insisted on deciphering my scribblings, typing them onto neat pages. Several years and drafts later, the story was taken in hand by Evelyn Monahan and Rosemary Neidel, and their masterful reworking of my text has brought the script to its finished state. To them I again extend my sincere thanks. A debt of gratitude is owed to Captain Lloyd G. Smith, OSS, and the family of Lieutenant Gary Duffy, British SOE, whose official reports documented our situation.

Preface

We are honored to help tell the story of a unique event in World War II history. The November 1943 crash-landing of a U.S. Army C-53—carrying thirteen army flight nurses, thirteen army medics, and a four-man flight crew—into Nazi-occupied Albania led to an amazing 800-mile walkout escape. That danger-filled journey took the group through enemy-held territory amid German troops and Nazi sympathizers, German bombing and strafing, and Ballist small-arms fire.

American military women were not supposed to be in combat areas or behind enemy lines, but, like the army nurses of Bataan and Corregidor who became prisoners of war in the Philippines, these thirteen flight nurses knew only too well that "supposed to be" had little to do with the actualities of military nursing during a world war.

Lieutenant Agnes Jensen and her colleagues had volunteered for the Army Nurse Corps and then for flight nurse training. They had already flown to the front lines and beyond to carry out their mission of nursing combat-wounded soldiers being transported to hospitals behind their own lines, knowing there was always the chance that the planes sent to collect the wounded would be shot down by the enemy, always the possibility of a crash behind enemy lines. Flight nurses knew these dangers before signing up for this pioneering venture in military nursing. Like Queen Esther of the Old Testament, they had answered their country's call and given action to her words: "I go, and if I perish, I perish."

Women's military history is an exciting and fertile field which has remained largely unexplored. Even a half-century after the end of World War II, many stories of courageous military women who served in every combat area remain untold. This book is offered to acquaint readers with one such story: the experiences of the U.S. Army flight nurses who made the astounding journey out of Nazi-occupied Albania.

In writing this history, we relied upon several primary sources. It is of couse, chiefly Agnes Jensen's view of events. Lieutenant Jensen kept a diary while on the ground in Albania and, after her return to safety, expanded her recollections in writing. Fortunately, she is still blessed with a memory of the smallest details of her life, such as the name of the ninth-grade teacher who taught her ancient history in a rural school in Michigan. Although the conversations quoted here cannot be said to be verbatim, they are as close as possible, given the documents available and Agnes Jensen Mangerich's excellent recall.

We also have used (and often present verbatim) the actual military reports of Lieutenant Gavin Duffy of the British Special Operations Executive (SOE) and Captain Lloyd Smith of the American Office of Strategic Services (OSS); U.S. Army Air Forces reports from the radio communications in Bari, Italy; military memoranda regarding the missing aircraft and search-and-rescue efforts; and a letter from T.E. Yarbrough, lead pilot of the three-aircraft mission.

The passengers and crew of Aircraft 42-68809, Sixty-first TC Sq, 314th TC Gp, were as follows:

Flight Nurses of the 807th Medical Air Evacuation Squadron

	Age	Hometown
2d Lt. Gertrude Dawson	29	Pittsburgh, Pennsylvania
2d Lt. Ann Maness	32	Paris, Texas
2d Lt. Jean Rutkowski	26	Detroit, Michigan
2d Lt. Elna Schwant	25	Winner, South Dakota
2d Lt. Lois Watson	25	Oaklawn, Illinois
2d Lt. Lillian Tacina	23	Hamtramck, Michigan
2d Lt. Pauleen Kanable	26	Richland Center, Wisconsin
2d Lt. Helen Porter	30	Hanksville, Utah
2d Lt. Ann Markowitz	25	Chicago, Illinois
2d Lt. Wilma Lytle	31	Butler, Kentucky
2d Lt. Frances Nelson	25	Princeton, West Virginia
2d Lt. Ann Kopsco	25	Hammond, Louisiana
2d Lt. Agnes Jensen	29	Stanwood, Michigan

Medics of the 807th Air Evacuation Squadron

T/Sgt. Lawrence O. Abbott	Newaygo, Michigan
T/Sgt. John P. Wolf	Milwaukee, Wisconsin
T/Sgt. Charles J. Adams	Niles, Michigan
T/Sgt. Robert A. Cranson	Sandy Creek, New York
T/Sgt. Raymond E. Eberg	Steeleville, Illinois
T/Sgt. Harold L. Hayes	Indianola, Iowa
T/Sgt. Robert E. Owen	Walden, New York
T/Sgt. Charles F. Zeiber	Reading, Pennsylvania
T/Sgt. Paul G. Allen	Greenville, Kentucky
T/Sgt. James P. Cruise	Brockton, Massachusetts
T/Sgt. William J. Eldridge	Eldridge, Kentucky
T/Sgt. Gordon M. MacKinnon	Los Angeles, California
Cpl. Hornsby (802d MAES)	Manchester, Kentucky

Flight Crew

Pilot: 1st Lt. Charles B. Thrasher	24	Daytona, Florida
Copilot: 2d Lt. James A. Baggs	28	Savannah, Georgia
Crew Chief: Sgt. Willis L. Shumway	23	Tempe, Arizona
Radio Operator: Sgt. Richard Lebo	24	Halifax, Pennsylvania

Introduction

Anyone stranded in Albania during World War II would confront not only inclement weather and rugged topography but the often brutal and intricate history of this occupied nation. It would be impossible to travel through the country without meeting its history head on. Certainly this was true for the members of a U.S. Army air crew and their passengers who crash-landed there in November 1943 and struggled for two months to reach the safety of the Allied lines.

At the geographical crossroads of many cultures, Albania has had a kaleidoscopic past, its borders, religions, and language altering in response to the aggressive treatment dealt by powerful, ambitious neighbors. First identified as a society of Bronze Age tribal people, the Albanians, fierce fighters, persevered through centuries of Greek and Roman domination, Byzantine rule, and wave after wave of invasions by Visigoths, Huns, Ostrogoths, Slavs, Serbs, and Normans. After nearly five centuries of Turkish governance, Albania emerged into the post–World War I era with a desire for self-rule but with a largely poverty-stricken, illiterate populace whose religious and tribal differences proved to be roadblocks to national unity and a peaceful coexistence.

Although Albania pronounced its independence in 1912, a viable national government eluded the best of plans throughout the Great War years. Foreign armies occupied or traveled across its territory at will. Greek and Italian intent to divide Albania, through the Secret Treaty of London in 1915, was thwarted by the Treaty of Versailles. This postwar pact upheld the ideal of Albanian autonomy, a principle strongly supported by U.S. President Woodrow Wilson. In 1919 Italy followed Greece in its withdrawal from Albania. When Albania was admitted to the League of Nations, the stage seemed to be set for the reestablishment of this beleaguered, war-weary country. Its effort at stability, however, was fraught with difficulties from the outset.

The new Albanian government was established at Tiranë in central Albania. Mendi Frasheri led the first Albanian delegation to the Paris Peace Conference. To the chagrin of those concerned, three other Albanian politicians also showed up, each claiming to be the head of the fledgling government. One of these impostors was assassinated in Paris at the instigation of the Italians, who considered him a troublemaker.

In the meantime, parts of Albania suffered continuing violence. In the northern part of the country the Serbs were attacking Albanians in retribution for prior Albanian onslaughts against them. In the southern province of Northern Epirus, Muslim Albanians were antagonizing and terrorizing their Christian neighbors, Albanians of Greek ancestry. In the town of Gjirokastër the Tiranian regime banned the Greek language, closed the private Greek schools, and sent barely literate Albanian priests to say the Mass in Albanian rather than in the traditional Greek. Easter Sunday 1921 ended in a riot when Albanian authorities seized the Archbishop of Korytsa and substituted an Albanian to perform the services. Another Greek priest was forced into a car, hustled across the border into Greece, and dumped off. As a result of such humiliations, pitched battles erupted between police and villagers. When the Northern Epirote Greeks sought the protection of the Serbian consul, they were advised that until the League of Nations took action, they should stay away from their schools and churches. As the flames of hatred were fanned, atrocities such as beatings and murder increased.

Actions by the League of Nations to quell the ethnic violence were largely ineffectual. When the League's Commission of Inquiry was sent to southern Albania in 1922 to investigate alleged atrocities, an unsavory Albanian who had served in the secret police and then as the nation's inspector of police accompanied the delegation, whose members were unaware that his presence made a farce of their inquiries.

Over the years Albania's boundaries, drawn and redrawn under innumerable treaties, were the cause of skirmishes and wars. In 1923, attempting to settle disputes over a section of the border with Greece, the League of Nations formed a Boundary Commission, which met a disastrous end. A chauffeur-driven car carrying the Italian members of the commission was blocked by a fallen tree and ambushed along an isolated stretch of road at the densely wooded Greek-Albanian frontier. Its passengers were mercilessly shot to death as they were trapped in the car or fled into the trees. The Albanian assassins escaped. Such incidents maintained Albania's chronic instability and failure to thrive as a nation.

Ideological divisions ran deep, creating cracks in a national armor already flawed by an all but bankrupt economy and a lack of effective national leadership. Amid government struggles with tribal uprisings and ethnic violence, however, a native Albanian who had been prominent in the now defunct Ottoman Empire gradually emerged to become minister of the interior, then president, and finally—as the potential democracy slid back into monarchy—as king. Ahmid Bey Zogu, an instrument of the Italian government, became King Zog and reigned from 1922 to 1939.

During that period Albania was tangled in a web of Yugoslavian and Italian intrigue, the results of which left the country in political and economic chaos. As Zog strove to unify Albania, he was bedeviled by attempts on his life, tribal revolts, and Italy's political and economic manipulations. He escaped several assassination attempts, once having to flee the country for his safety. But he was soon returned to the throne by the Italians, who had much to gain from his powerful position. In exchange for a series of unsolicited loans, for example, the Italian banks demanded securities in the form of Albanian mineral and forestry rights. When the "borrowers" defaulted, as the lenders had known they would, the Italian demands for reparation functioned to drain this economically anemic country of such natural resources as oil, fisheries, and lumber.

Meanwhle, Zog dealt with internal uprisings through the time-honored Albanian practice of attacking and executing the rebels and burning their villages, and by the banishment of arms, a prohibition introduced during the Ottoman rule. Censorship was enforced on various matters, including discussions on the controversial issue of closing the Greek schools.

Still, Zog had a few inclinations toward democracy. These included sporadically announced elections and his interest in emancipating women from the repressive Muslim code of face covering. In 1937 he pronounced a new law that sanctioned punishment of Muslim and Christian women for wearing veils, and made marriage and divorce civil rather than religious matters.

Zog's reign was nevertheless strewn with blatant examples of partiality in favor of Muslims, a historic Ottoman double standard of justice in legal matters both civil and criminal. The Christians, frequently the victims of crimes, were particularly outraged when known murderers were allowed to go unpunished. Such inequities acted like gasoline on the already blazing fires of hatred and caused the Greek government in 1935 to request intervention by the League of Nations on the closing of Greek schools. Since the matter was covered in the minorities declaration that had been signed by Albania in 1922 as a prerequisite for admission to the League, Albania's representative had little recourse but to tell the League that the school-closing dilemma would be rectified. Albania was granted three months to comply. The feudal Muslim leaders, meeting in Gjirokastër, proposed a plan to expel the Albanian-Greek peasants and allow the land to be taken over by Muslims, thus ridding Albania of (in their eyes) undesirable Christians. The plan was rejected as threatening economic catastrophe, since the industrious Christians paid significant sums in taxes to the Albanian government. To relieve the pressure brought by the League, the Albanians sent erroneous proof that the Greek private schools had been reopened. This further fed long-standing hatreds and created an environment for continuing confrontation and violence.

In 1938 the armaments necessary for a national defense against the modern-day Hun and his fascist Italian counterpart, Hitler and Mussolini, were nonexistent. Albania was technologically, economically, and psychologically unprepared for any foreign aggression. When Mussolini invaded in April 1939 the previously intrepid King Zog fled to England, and the Albanians offered little resistance to the invasion from across the Adriatic Sea. Once again an occupied nation, the Albanians positioned themselves for survival by using the ancient, proven practice of withdrawing to the higher, more protected mountains and developing a variety of resistance movements, which formed along ideological lines. Three major forces—mutual enemies—formed as first the Italians and then the Germans invaded Albania.

The Albanian National Liberation Front of the Communist Party (LNC) was instigated by Tito, who founded the Yugoslavian LNC when Hitler invaded Russia. Early in 1943 Tito named Enver Hoxa, a Muslim from Gjirokastër, as a "Colonel-General" in the Albanian LNC, with instructions to organize citizens into a guerrilla movement against impending Nazi invasion. The LNC, whose base of operation was constantly on the move, had one goal: to harass the occupying Germans by destroying their supplies and striking them sporadically when they least expected it, in an effort to demoralize their personnel and weaken their impact. The LNC's methods were familiar to Albanians, who had survived centuries of foreign occupation by employing similar tactics. The LNC was supplied with weapons, ammunition, and other necessities by the British and Americans during World War II.

Second, the Northern Epirote National Liberation Organization (EAOBH) was a local resistance group, a branch of the Greek National Democratic League (EDES). The Albanian leader was Basil Sachines from the village of Douvini. An outspoken, prosperous businessman in Gjirokastër, he became targeted by the Albanian police for his support of Albanian-Greek citizens. He was assassinated by the LNC on November 17, 1943. Two military officers led other sections of the Northern Epirote resistance movement, Spyridon Litos and John Videles, who was also the liaison to the EDES. Their headquarters moved from place to place in southern Albania.

Third, the Balli Kombetar was a counterresistance group organized to support an Albanian fascist militia. By arming small groups of citizens to fight local guerrillas, the Italians and then the Germans and the militia were free to concentrate on other concerns. The Ballists were cofounded by Ali Klisura and Midhat Bey Frasheri, the first president of this group and son of Abdyl Bey Frasheri, who had participated in the 1878 Congress of Prizren which sought to keep Albania in the Ottoman Empire. The son's political career be-

gan in the Young Turk Party, which mounted a revolution in 1909
aimed at salvaging the waning Ottoman rule. Under Frasheri's leadership, the Ballists were well supplied by the Nazis. They received
thousands of guns and 600,000 napoleons, equivalent to 12 million
gold francs. The Balli Kombetar had its headquarters in Nazi-occupied Tiranë.

The British Mission, under the Special Operations Executive
(SOE), a branch of British army intelligence, had arrived in Albania
by early 1943 to work with the LNC and the Greek guerrilla movements. Anticipating the surrender of Italy to the Allies in September
1943 and the subsequent withdrawal of Italian troops from Albania,
the British foresaw an escalation in Ballist activities under the Nazis.
Thus they proposed that the EAOBH and the LNC (partisans) col-
laborate to form a stronger force against the Germans and the Balli
Kombetar, and arranged for several meetings near Gjirokastër in
August and September 1943. Negotiations were difficult, crippled
by mutual distrust and deep-seated hatreds between the two groups,
which had only months before been engaged in a fierce battle at
Liskovic on the Greek-Albanian frontier. Their collaborative efforts
were only moderately and spasmodically successful.

In July 1943 the German Army F and the 100th Light Division, commanded by General Alexander Loehr, arrived in Albania.
They were blocked, but only temporarily, by the LNC, which had
seized the Tiranë airfield. In October the Germans mounted a major offensive in Northern Epirus and fierce fighting occurred between the EAOBH and a combined force of Ballists, Albanian fascist
militia, and Nazis. The results were devastating. As the Italian troops
retreated, many had looted and burned villages in their paths; now
the Ballists and Germans attacked Epirote villages, putting the inhabitants to death by firing squads, despite gender or age; burning
the houses, some of which were locked with their occupants inside;
and hanging the village priests.

By November the Germans were in firm control in Albania.
On the 8th—the day the U.S. Army plane carrying the 807th Medical Air Evacuation Unit crash-landed—a formal puppet government
was installed in Tiranë, and troop strength had been increased. In
December, Germany had 700,000 troops in the Balkans. German

infantry squads set up a network of checkpoints, at approximately six-mile intervals, to protect roads and bridges against guerrilla assaults. In the south the Ballists controlled most parts of Northern Epirus.

In 1943 Albania was considered the poorest, most backward country in Europe. Three-quarters of its 11,110 square miles is rugged mountainous terrain, from which cascade five major rivers that can become raging torrents and flood the narrow coastal plain from November through March. Julius Caesar in 48 B.C. commented in his journal that the river crossings were major obstacles for his Roman army. Along the low and hazardous coastline there was only one safe cove and one natural harbor, both under Nazi control in the winter of 1943-44. With only twenty-six miles of paved roads in Albania, most people traveled by foot or pack animal. Few homes had electricity or indoor plumbing, and food was scarce. For the 807th Medical Air Evacuation Unit personnel, who had set out on a routine mission, their unplanned descent into Albania must have seemed like dropping through a tear in the curtain of time.

1 Crash Landing

8 November 1943, Monday—0745: Catania, Sicily

A cold drizzle was falling when the jeeps carrying thirteen U.S. Army nurses and twelve medical technical sergeants of the 807th Medical Air Evacuation Squad (MAES), plus one young corporal with the 802d MAES who was catching a ride back to his assigned base, pulled onto the apron of a runway at Catania Main Airfield in Sicily. They stopped alongside a C-53, one of the three aircraft that would make up the flight scheduled to carry them the 260 miles to Bari, Italy, to pick up wounded and fly them to hospitals farther behind the lines.

Winter weather in the Mediterranean was frequently dangerous, and bad weather had canceled the flight twice in the last two days. Today's weather report was predicting a serious storm moving in from the north, but all reasonable calculations said the flight would be in Bari at least two hours before the storm struck along their flight path.

Second Lieutenant Agnes A. Jensen was the first to board the plane. She walked forward, placed her musette bag in the first bucket seat and sat down in the second. The first seat on the right-hand side was not a good place to sit because several knobs connected to the radio protruded into the space at head level.

The other twelve nurses piled their gear in the front seat and sat down on the same side of the plane. Sergeant Paul Allen, a medic from her unit, sat opposite Lieutenant Jensen, and a young corporal she did not recognize took the seat diagonally across from her. The rest of the men filled in.

The pilots stepped through the door and stopped to talk with Captain Robert Simpson, a squadron doctor who had accompanied the nurses to the plane. Simpson was waiting for final word concerning the weather before he and the jeeps returned to the 807th billeting area.

In the two months the 807th had been overseas, they had flown with different pilots, on any plane they could catch, on their way to pick up wounded GIs. Medical Air Evacuation was so new that no planes were actually assigned to the medical squadrons. The 314th Troop Carrier Group ferried troops, medical personnel, and patients around the Mediterranean Theater of Operations, and within the group the Fifty-second Troop Carrier Wing made frequent trips through Catania Main to various locations in Italy. Nurses and medical technicians caught rides to collecting areas where they would be split into teams and assigned to various planes carrying patients to hospitals in the theater.

Lieutenant Jensen registered the fact that she and her squad had not previously flown with either of the two pilots standing in the aisle of the C-53. The senior pilot, a slim, dark-haired first lieutenant, was speaking to Captain Simpson.

"The weather report says there's a cold front moving down from Naples, but we should be in Bari hours ahead of it. So, we're on our way."

He and the copilot, a second lieutenant with reddish blond hair, walked up the aisle and disappeared into the cockpit.

Jensen and the other nurses were getting magazines and hometown newspapers from coat pockets and fastening their seat belts when Captain Simpson paused at the door of the plane and called, "Good luck, gang!" With a playful smile he added, "Any last words, kids? Any messages you want sent home?"

Everyone laughed and someone called back, "Just spread the word—keep 'em flying!"

The door of the plane closed and it taxied to the runway. It was 0815 hours as the plane left the ground and began the journey that would carry those on board into one of the most remarkable experiences of World War II.

Lieutenant Jensen loved being an army flight nurse. Takeoff

was especially exciting to her. She liked the roar of the engines as the plane actually lifted off the runway and the ground slipped away beneath them. It was as if she were being freed from earthly matters and everyday routine. She watched out a window as the rugged Sicilian terrain flattened and was replaced by the Mediterranean Sea. But the usually brilliant blue water was an ominous dark green, flecked everywhere with frothy white. Ugly dark clouds loomed off to the left, and the air was becoming rougher with each passing minute.

Probably a local thunderstorm, Lieutenant Jensen thought. We should be able to skirt its edges. There was nothing unusual about a thunderstorm in this area, and the squad had flown around a dozen of them in the past two months.

Might as well read a little, Jensen thought. She picked up her magazine and tried to make out the words in the dim light filtering through the plane's windows.

"Have you been to Naples yet?" Jensen looked up from her article and saw the round face and short hair of Elna Schwant, a twinkle in her green eyes. "That's where I'd like to go next," Elna said. "How about you, Jens?"

"Naples would be swell," Jens said. "But I think the 802d considers it their territory. They've pretty much claimed the entire west coast."

"Well, Ann Maness just got back from Naples recently," Elna said. "She loved the place."

"That was on a specially requested plane," Jens said. "We don't get too many requests like that. Besides, according to Ann, there was an air raid or two on the field every night. Not to mention that the dogfights seemed to take place exclusively over the nurses' quarters. But she did manage to get to Pompeii in the one-day layover." Jens felt her own excitement. As a child of Danish immigrant parents, she had dreamed of traveling to foreign places ever since she could remember. When she completed nursing school, she had applied for a nursing position with a Swedish-American steamship line, but her hopes were dashed with the application's second question, "Which languages do you speak?" Her parents had never taught her their native tongue, and that job application caused her to regret the fact deeply. Her search for adventure in faraway places led her next to the U.S. Army Nurse Corps, which she joined in February 1941, before America entered World War II. "I can't wait to see it for myself. Pompeii, Rome, Florence, Milan. Sometimes I can't believe how lucky I was to get this assignment."

"Lucky?" Elna demanded.

"Yeah. I just knew that our training in the heat of Louisville was to condition us for service on New Guinea."

Without warning the plane was suddenly jolted by violent buffeting. It seemed to stand on end, then flip from side to side so quickly that Jens was surprised they were still right-side up. She pulled her seat belt tighter, looked out the window, and saw the wings flapping frantically, as if they were trying to get someone's attention. Jens had never seen wings flap so hard and fast and silently said a prayer that they had been constructed with this kind of weather in mind. The planes were in the middle of the storm, and even a novice knew this was not a good place to be.

Jens turned her back to the window and opened her magazine. We'll be through this soon, she assured herself. It was too dark to read so she turned her thoughts to Bari and tried to remember what her ninth-grade teacher of ancient history, Mr. DisBrow, had taught about it.

Certainly Bari, Brindisi, and all the east coast of Italy were very much a part of that old civilization. Her teacher had given her the impression that this part of Europe was not relevant in today's world. It sure seems important at the moment, Jens told herself.

Lights came on in the plane, but they didn't help reading one bit. The violent dropping and flopping were so constant and fierce that only their seat belts kept them from piling out into the aisle or hitting the ceiling.

Nurses and medics had been trained too well to allow what they felt internally to be reflected on their faces. Fear and panic were contagious, and medical personnel were determined not to start or feed either.

Tremendous drops were accompanied by horrendous cracking noises throughout the plane. Then the cabin would be filled with the sounds of sudden crashes as the floor caught up with loose equipment when they were suddenly thrust upward.

Jens tried to read again but was unable to form the separate words into intelligible sentences. I can't do a thing about the weather, she told herself. I'll just have to trust the two pilots, whoever they are!

0840: Cockpit of Lead Aircraft

First Lieutenant T.E. Yarbrough, pilot in the lead aircraft, remained in frequent contact with the two other planes in the flight. Visibility was deteriorating rapidly, and before ordering the flight to go on instruments Yarbrough radioed Lieutenant Charles B. Thrasher, flying off his right wing, to descend 500 feet, and Lieutenant Joseph Rogers, off his left wing, to climb 500 feet. Yarbrough ordered the planes to accomplish the separation by performing a 360-degree turn while changing altitude. The end result was a separation of five to ten miles between aircraft. Yarbrough's plane continued at the planned altitude of 8,000 feet with Thrasher now at 7,500 feet and Rogers at 8,500.

The weather was continuing to worsen, and Yarbrough noticed he was picking up ice on his wings. He immediately radioed to Thrasher and Rogers to use their de-ice boots. The three planes maintained radio contact until they reached the outskirts of Bari.

0855: Cabin of Lieutenant Thrasher's Aircraft

Despite the downdrafts, it was evident from the increasing cold that they were gaining altitude. The metal bucket seats transferred the cold with a vengeance. Jens raised up slightly and slid a magazine between herself and the seat. The plane was uninsulated, and the cabin was fast becoming like the inside of a refrigerator. The turbulence was growing worse. The plane lurched, stood on end for a second, then plummeted downward, bucking all the way. Suddenly it was much warmer and brighter inside the cabin, and Jens thought the worst was over. That happy thought lasted only long enough for her to glance out the window and see that they were nearly skimming the water. A frightening thought flashed across her mind. My God! Are they ditching without a word of warning? We must be in real trouble. What about life rafts and life jackets? She couldn't remember seeing any rafts on board, but she had spotted about ten

Mae Wests swinging from a cable in the rear of the plane. She did a little math in her head: ten Mae Wests, twenty-six people in the cabin and four flight crew in the cockpit.

Jens's eyes remained frozen on the water as Elna looked out the same window. Neither betrayed in word or gesture what they were feeling. Their training as flight nurses had taken over automatically.

Suddenly they were climbing again, and Jens felt relieved that they weren't ditching—not yet anyway.

She thought of her previous two flights. Both had taken place in clear weather and had terminated on the airfield at Grottaglie. Today they were to overfly Grottaglie and go straight to Bari. They would probably be a little late, Jens told herself; after all, the head winds are pretty strong.

The plane banked sharply, and Jens realized they were flying in circles. She looked at her watch. It was 1000 hours, and she reasoned that they must be over Bari, but it would take some time to let down in this murky weather. The circling continued and so did the violent downdrafts. Another downdraft like that last one, and we'll be on the ground faster than anyone hoped.

The door to the cockpit popped open, and the radio operator walked directly to the first bucket seat. He gave the protruding radio knobs a turn or two, took some equipment from the bulkhead next to Jens, and returned to the cockpit. The door didn't close completely, and the passengers could see him working frantically with the radio.

That's all we need in this weather—no radio, Jens told herself. One of the cockpit crew pulled the door closed. They continued to fly in circles.

We're already overdue, Jens thought. We must be over Bari. Maybe they're having trouble contacting the ground at the base. They continued to fly in circles.

1031: Cockpit of Thrasher's Aircraft

At 1031 Thrasher contacted the base station at Bari and asked for the weather report. The station challenged Thrasher, requesting the password of the day, but he was unable to provide it. Consequently the information he requested was not given to him.

At 1050 he made contact again and asked that the beacon be turned on. Again he was unable to answer the challenge, and the beacon was not turned on. At 1100 Thrasher asked for the beacon again, and for the third time was unable to provide the password. The beacon was not turned on. At 1135 he asked to be given a radio fix, but the station did not have the necessary equipment. At 1145 the radio beacon was turned on for ten minutes even though Thrasher was still unable to identify himself with the password. After 1155 the radio station in Bari was unable to make contact with Thrasher.

1156: Cabin of Thrasher's Aircraft

The plane had stopped flying in circles and was flying straight again. Jens hoped the pilots knew what they were doing—had they missed Bari? Were they unable to make contact because the radio wasn't working? Were they headed for an alternate airfield? But there were no other airfields available to them in southern Italy.

The plane flew on for a long time. For a moment the air cleared, and Jens could see that they were high above water. Elna nudged her and pointed to two water spouts skipping over the surface. The two watched until lack of visibility sealed them inside the plane again.

The turbulence had let up considerably, and the plane flew in and out of clouds, every now and then allowing them a glimpse of the sea beneath.

The cabin temperature had dropped further, and Jens slid a second magazine between herself and the metal seat. She glanced at the other passengers in the cabin. Most were watching intently out their windows; others were attempting to read, trying to close out the reality of the situation.

"Mountains?" Elna asked, and pointed out the window. Her bright green eyes and smile said she was happy with the world.

She can't be that happy about being over mountains, Jens thought. In an instant she remembered that Elna smiled almost perpetually, no matter what reality she was facing.

Jens looked out the window. There were mountains all right. Rugged, jagged peaks sticking up out of the clouds.

"Where do you think we are?" Elna asked.

"There are mountains in southern Italy at the toe, but there are also mountains in northern Italy," Jens said.

"Maybe they're returning to Sicily," Elna said.

"I don't know," Jens said. She shrugged. "About the only thing I do know is that I'm freezing." She pulled her feet up, wrapped her coat around her legs, and sat huddled with her chin on her knees.

Suddenly she was very aware of the young sergeant seated across from her. He was shaking all over and had bent down and clasped his arms around his knees in an effort to hold them still. At first Jens thought that he must be even colder than she was, but the look on his face changed her mind. He's shaking with fear, she thought. With his turned-up nose and shock of brown hair sticking out from under his knit olive drab cap he looked as young as her seventeen-year-old brother. Watching him, she became aware of her own fears. She leaned forward and looked down the line of nurses, sitting in those bucket seats, facing the aisle with stoic expressions. Each nurse had mastered the self-discipline taught at air evacuation school.

There were several loud clanks as ice came off the wings and was blown against the fuselage. The dark-haired pilot popped through the cockpit door just as the clanking became louder and more frequent. He looked excited.

"We can see a field and we're going to try for it," he said. "It might be rough, so buckle up."

"A field?" one of the nurses said.

"An airfield?" a sergeant asked.

It was 1210 and they were long overdue at Bari. Twenty-six people squirmed to look out the windows.

Jens could see a large hole in the clouds, and through it she glimpsed the ground below. They were descending very fast. For the first time in hours an excited chatter filled the cabin. A man's voice at the rear of the plane boomed above the rest.

"Yup, yup, a real airfield. Anyway there are planes on it."

Jens couldn't see the field, but what she could see was not encouraging. Several black puffs of smoke rose and billowed just in front of the propellers and near each wing as the plane pitched erratically. There was a clanking sound on the fuselage at the rear, and all twenty-six people looked toward the tail—then stared at each other as the aircraft began to climb steeply into the clouds. The radioman came out of the cockpit and peered through the windows on both sides of the plane before looking at the passengers.

"That was close! That was a German field we damn near landed on. Did you see that ack-ack? Deadly accurate stuff," he said.

"So that's what the clanking on the tail was?" the young corporal asked.

Without another word the radioman disappeared into the cockpit. The excited comments dwindled, then died out completely. For the first time, the truth and seriousness of their situation loomed in front of Jens.

"Did you see those two Messerschmitts?" a sergeant asked. "They're following to shoot us down."

Jens watched out a window as the plane entered a thick cloud bank. My God, she thought, we've been flying for four hours, and the pilots don't even know where we are. If that was a German field, we must be over northern Italy. What are they doing heading even farther north? I thought we circled Bari, but I must have been wrong. Why would they fly north if they reached Bari?

The Allied armistice with the Italians had been signed on 3 September 1943, only sixty-six days earlier, but German troops were still firmly in control of northern Italy, and no doubt many bloody battles still stood between this day and an Italy in Allied hands. In the past lay Salerno and the fighting in a hundred small towns where Allied soldiers breathed their last and now slept beneath the rows of silent white crosses left behind.

Thrasher's plane was surely in unfriendly territory, but where, and how far from Allied lines?

Another series of clanks beat on the fuselage as ice lifted off the wings, and Jens felt relieved that the de-icers were working. She remembered having once said she would never bail out unless both engines were on fire, but this seemed a perfect time to reassess her position. She wished she had a parachute so she would have a chance to make the decision for herself. The new parachutes with which they had each been so carefully fitted, stenciled with their names like all their other flying clothes, had been sent ahead from the States with the squadron's equipment but never arrived, or at least were never found. Someone, somewhere, somehow had made the decision that they could fly without them. Evidently someone had concluded that since patients wouldn't have parachutes, nurses didn't need them either. Jens had a persistent feeling that although air evacuation was trying to prove itself, nurses were expendable.

Anyway, here they were, but where? A horrible thought filled her mind: there was not one soul on the plane who knew.

Looking out the window, she could see that they were flying at about the same altitude as the mountain peaks jabbing up through the clouds. Wham! Everything on the plane clattered as they flopped dizzily for a few seconds during a rough downdraft. The engines sounded as if the wind had almost blown them out and they were trying hard to catch up again. Was it the wind or the altitude that made them gasp? Jens's feet felt like ice, and she pulled them up and wrapped her coat around them for the second time.

It was nearly 1300, and their aircraft had been buffeted about for five hours. Jens was certain that she had forgotten what a smooth flight was like. There had been no further communication from the cockpit, and all chatter had died in the cabin.

Jens examined the faces of the sergeants. Most of them looked very concerned, if not outright scared. No wonder, she thought. We seem to have only two options: hit one of the mountain peaks, or run out of gas and crash. Neither was very comforting. Jens decided to do what she could. She straightened out the musette bags on the seat next to her, making a sort of mound. She loosened her seat belt, slid down, and placed her head on the makeshift pillow. Sleep had always come easily to her, and she hoped it wouldn't desert her now. She felt terribly weary and strangely relieved as she closed her eyes. She couldn't shut out the roar of the motors, but she converted it to a constant hum and drifted off to sleep.

Jens awakened to the pilot's voice before she actually saw him standing in the cockpit door.

"We are going to land," he announced.

"Where?" the question rose as from one voice.

His only response was, "And buckle up tight because this time it's wheels up and it will be rough." He disappeared into the cockpit.

Jens turned to Elna to get information she was sure she'd missed while sleeping. "Where are we going to land?" Jens asked.

"On the ground, I hope," Elna said with a toothy grin.

For a moment Jens wanted to hit her but decided against it. She squirmed to get a better look out the window. Through a hole in the clouds, she could see flat land. They were losing altitude fast by making a very tight turn down through the opening. Jens pulled her seat belt tighter and looked at the young sergeant. He had stopped shaking and was tightening his seat belt and staring straight ahead.

The extreme turns were making Jens dizzy and had left her stomach in the clouds. Glancing at the radio knobs and buttons on the bulkhead, she placed her head on her knees and wrapped her arms firmly around her legs. One lesson from the survival course surfaced, and she repeated it silently to herself. There are usually two jolts in a crash landing, whether on land or on water, so keep your seat belt fastened until you are reasonably sure that the aircraft has come to a stop. But once it has, clear out quickly. Planes don't usually float very long, and on land there is always a good chance of fire and explosion.

Jens braced herself, interpreting the sounds of the motors to mean that a crash landing was imminent. To her delight, the plane touched down and was rolling. Thank God, she thought, the wheels are down. She tried to raise her head and found that the plane's momentum had her pinned in place. The same force caused the line of nurses beside her to slip forward, pressing their weight against Jens, and she, against the bags and equipment in the first bucket seat.

In a split second the plane stopped abruptly, the tail flipped upward, and the nose buried itself in the ground.

2 On the Ground

8 November 1943, Monday—1340: On the Ground in Enemy Territory

There was a thunderous clash and clatter as everything that was not tied down in the tail of the aircraft, flew forward. Jens raised her head slightly and saw that the crew chief was sprawled in the aisle, along with ration cans, tins of drinking water, cardboard boxes, and a myriad of smaller objects. A strong jolt shook the plane as the tail settled back down, and one of the crew raced to open the door.

Everyone bolted into action and tried to pile out all at once until a nurse in the rear yelled, "Now just a minute! Have you lost your minds? Pick up that man."

Her command had a sobering effect. A couple of the men reached down, picked up the crew chief without changing stride, and went quickly out the door.

Jens was one of the last people off and discovered there was no need for the ladder; the ground was even with the door. She stepped out into a fine drizzling rain and sank immediately into mud that got deeper and more slippery with every step. Looking around, she realized that they had landed in a field of corn stubble.

It was a desolate spot in a fairly wide valley; high mountains on both sides cut off any view of what might lie beyond them. We must be miles from nowhere, Jens thought, as her feet continued to sink in the mushy earth. She started toward the front of the plane to see what damage had been done to the nose and props. Movement around trees and bushes on the side of the mountain facing them, stopped her in her tracks. As she watched intently, she could make out people running toward them. As they got closer, Jens could see that they were men of short stature, slight build, and dark complexion. They had rifles slung on their backs, and the weapons bounced up and down as they ran. Some wore white fezzes and others had dull blue uniform caps. The first man to reach the downed aircraft rode astride a large white horse. He had a black cape flowing behind him, a rifle on his back, and a double row of ammunition on a diagonal belt across his chest; hand grenades hung from his waist. A large black mustache accented a wide smile that showed most of his tobacco-stained teeth. He dismounted immediately. Jens was so engrossed with this horseman's appearance that at first she didn't see his outstretched hand. The man had a booming voice. "Americano! Americano!" he shouted. He grabbed Jens's right hand and shook it for almost a full minute.

"Where are we? Italy?" Jens asked. She pointed at him. "Italiano?" she asked.

"No, no!" he said and arched backward. He seemed displeased at the inference. He pointed to his cap. It had a double eagle in black on a red background, with a red star above. "Russia. Russia," he repeated, rolling his Rs with linguistic perfection.

Jens felt her eyes pop and her mouth fly open. "But," she stammered, "we can't be in Russia. We were just over water an hour ago. Or could we be? Did I sleep that long?"

Without replying, the man in the black cape moved on to other members of the party and was briskly shaking their hands.

Jens watched with amazement as the rest of the people approached. They wore black trousers of a coarse hand-woven wool material with tight-fitting legs laced up the sides. Knee-length capes of the same cloth, some white but most black, were flung over their shoulders. A few had good leather shoes that looked English, but most had pieces of kidskin that scarcely covered their toes and reached about an inch above the sole of the foot all the way around. These were held in place by kidskin thongs that crisscrossed over the instep, were caught once just over the toe and heel and twice on either side, then tied around the ankles, which were well protected from the cold weather by heavy hand-knit wool socks.

Her companions from the plane were walking around in a semi-dazed state. Jens watched them for a moment. "We're all here," she said. "We all made it." She felt weak with relief.

Suddenly the blond copilot dashed around the wing of the plane. "We're in Albania. One of these men speaks a little English. He says the Germans are close by. So get your gear. Hurry! We have to leave now. They may have seen or heard us come down."

The Americans rushed into the plane as quickly as they had left it moments ago. The aisle was crowded with dislodged cargo: K rations, pint tins of emergency water, three life rafts, five parachutes, three GI blankets, a fleece-lined flight suit. Several sergeants unscrewed a section of bucket seats to use as a stretcher for the injured crew chief, while the rest of the party grabbed whatever they could carry.

Outside, the medics placed the injured man on the makeshift stretcher while several of the Albanians relieved the others of portions of their load and indicated by motions that the foreign visitors should follow them in a quick dogtrot. They jogged off in a loose formation, making their way through a muddy field that was dotted with low, scrubby bushes and high coarse grass. In a matter of minutes their clean, well-pressed army uniforms were splattered with mud, and the bottoms of their slacks were sopping wet.

Rain had turned the uphill trail into a slippery, tiring challenge. The men took turns carrying the crew chief's stretcher, and several helped steady those bearing the load. Despite the conditions, the party agreed, they were lucky to have survived the German ack-ack earlier and now the crash landing. Jens was surprised to see the blond-haired pilot riding the white horse at the front of this procession. That horse is probably a lot more surefooted than the rest of us, she thought, as she pulled one foot after the other out of the mud and fought her way uphill. After more than an hour she spotted a building in the distance and hoped it was their destination. Every step introduced her to a new muscle and reminded her that she didn't get much exercise. She breathed in the cold, wet air and pushed ahead.

The thirty survivors had been walking for two hours when they arrived at a small, squat stone house. Overlapping slabs of rock covered the roof and glistened in the rain. They followed their Albanian escorts up an outside staircase to the second floor and into a small smoky room. A dirty woolen rug, handmade and once white, covered most of the area around an oblong open hearth that protruded almost to the middle of the room. Two small windows with sagging shutters closed out the light but not the weather. A smoldering fire had filled the room with smoke. All thirty Americans and four Albanians crowded into the room and squatted around the fire, peeling off their wet outer garments.

Lois Watson sat next to Jens and held up a small mirror to look at a gash on her cheek. Jens examined the cut, which was swollen and caked with blood.

"Does it hurt much?" Jens asked.

"No, not really, but something must have hit me hard because a few of my teeth are loose," Lois answered.

"What hit you, do you know?" Jens asked.

"The only thing I remember flying through the air was the crew chief," Lois laughed.

Fran Nelson, a brown-eyed brunette with fine-boned features who was sitting on the other side of Lois, leaned forward. "His foot just missed the end of my nose as he went past me," she said.

"Oh," said Lois. "I'll just bet his foot caught me on the cheek. I do remember trying to look quickly at the rear of the plane. I probably stuck my head out far enough for his shoe to hit me. It all went so quickly at the end." She pushed her blond hair back, and Jens could see her round blue eyes above the welt on her cheek.

"The Krauts were deadly accurate with that ack-ack over their field. I looked at the tail of the plane after we got out; it had shrapnel holes in it. That's what that clunking was that we heard," said a dark young man with a medium build and thin mustache. Jens noticed three stripes on his sleeve and knew he was a buck sergeant. All the medical sergeants had three stripes with two rocker stripes added.

"You must be the radioman. I remember seeing you working on it," Jens said.

"That's right. Dick Lebo is my name."

Jens introduced herself, then asked, "What happened? Why did we miss Bari so completely?"

"I'm not sure we missed it. I thought we contacted the tower.

We gave the usual message and then asked for instructions, but before we heard anything, the radio quit." He nodded toward the wounded crew chief and went on. "Shumway and I worked on it, but couldn't get another sound out of it. Flames were shooting down the companionway from the antennae earlier, when we were in that thunderstorm, so maybe that's what finished it."

"Just where in Albania are we? Do you have any idea?" Jens asked.

"Near Yugoslavia. Does that help?"

"How many miles of water would you guess at its narrowest spot to Italy?" asked a young-faced sergeant with steel-rimmed glasses.

"Ninety to a hundred miles maybe, from the southern part of Albania to Bari or Brindisi," Lebo said.

"I see no possibility of getting that plane out, do you?" the round-faced sergeant asked.

"No, and the props are all bent," Lebo said quietly.

Still others joined their conversation. They talked of walking to the coast and the possibility, once there, of getting a boat large enough to hold all thirty of them. They speculated that there might be a big sailboat like the fishing boats they used to buzz, along the coast of Sicily.

The sergeant with the glasses said he used to sail a little, and the group turned toward him.

"Oh, good," Lois said. "There must be boats along the shore."

They had been absorbed in their conversation for hours. It was not until someone opened the door that Jens realized it had grown dark outside. She noticed Elna staring at the fire. "What are you dreaming about?"

"Any dreams better come equipped with wings and motors." It was voice of the young corporal who had sat diagonally across the aisle from Jens. His mischievous smile and remark made everyone laugh with relief.

"I was wondering if Captain Voight was out to meet our plane in Bari today and how long he waited for us," Elna said.

"Do you suppose anyone is aware yet that we didn't land at any field in Italy?" Fran asked.

"If the weather was this stinko all over, they probably weren't expecting us at all," Lois said.

Things were quiet for about ten minutes. Ann "Marky" Markowitz, a twenty-five-year-old nurse whose hometown was Chicago, suddenly popped up with, "Do you realize that this is half our 807th squadron right here—half of the flight personnel, I should say."

"Do you realize I didn't have to come today?" Jean Rutkowski asked. Jean was a former airline stewardess from Detroit.

"Oh, no, what happened?" Elna asked.

"Stakeman counted wrong and added one too many, and when it wasn't noticed till this morning, I decided I might as well go on to Italy, because half the battle is getting up at 5 A.M. At least that's what I thought then. So here I am, lucky me!"

"I'm glad now that I was CQ, Charge of Company Quarters, yesterday," Jens said, "because I wrote several letters home, so it will be a month or more before they get too concerned about my not writing."

"A month!" Fran exclaimed. "We can't—I brought only one change of clothes this trip, and my gosh, no shampoo."

Lois nudged her. "I can think of something more important I didn't bring."

Fran clapped her hands over her mouth as she gasped again. "I didn't bring any either."

It wasn't yet 2100, but sleep was overtaking the party one by one. All of them had been up since 0500, and it had been a trying and stressful day. Jens shifted her position in the small space she had, and her legs felt five feet long. "What time did we land, does anyone know?"

"Between 1300 and 1330," the blond pilot answered in a Georgia drawl. In the firelight his face looked redder and his eyebrows and eye lashes lighter.

"Weren't you riding that white horse up the trail?" Jens asked him.

He nodded. "He belongs to our friend here." He patted the knee of the man seated next to him.

"Yes, my horse," said the Albanian in English.

The pilot introduced him. "This is Hassan, didn't you see him before?"

"Yes," said Jens. "I talked with you at the plane. You have a very beautiful horse."

"Yes," he said. "He very good horse, that horse. He may keep you from being shooted today."

"Shooted?" Jens asked. "How is that?"

"Well, after plane stop we think, of course, it is Germani, but one young boy standing by me say, 'No, not Germani, because it has star.' So I ride out on my horse very fast." He took a deep breath and, wagging his finger for emphasis, added, "Because if I no come fast with my white horse, the partisans who come very fast to greet you, would shoot you one and one and one as you come from plane." He motioned like shooting and laughed as though it were a joke. "That is why I make Meester Baggs ride horse. Just friends ride my horse."

Baggs laughed. "No wonder he pushed me back on the animal; I wanted to get off so someone else could ride, but he insisted that I stay on."

"You're the copilot, right?" Jens asked.

"Yes, I'm Jim Baggs."

"I'm Jens. Just half of my last name, Jensen. What happened to us today? Did we come out over Bari? Lebo thought you'd contacted them."

He threw up his hands, looked across the fire, and said, "I'm not sure." He continued looking away, and then began talking to Hassan. Jens thought of a lot of questions to ask them, but was too weary to pursue the matter at that moment and instead, asked how Shumway, the injured crew chief, was doing.

Ann Kopsco, a former stewardess with Delta Airlines, pulled herself up on one elbow. "We cleaned up his knee, nothing seems to be broken, and he's had some morphine. We've got his leg elevated, but with no ice to reduce the swelling, he'll be limping for a while."

Most of the group had already settled back on the crowded floor, and exhaustion had pushed them into sleep. Jens explored her possible sleeping space and discovered the most she could claim allowed her to lean back a bit in the space where she was sitting. In the five and a half hours they had been in this small smoky room, they had not been offered food or water. The men who had brought in firewood hours earlier had not reappeared. Her best guess was that they were with partisans and were in one of their hideouts. In the middle of a war, she thought, we've managed to land in a country that's been in a civil war for years. Oh, well, it's a lot better than not walking away from a crash landing. Her mind filled with images and memories of her survival training at Bowman Field, Kentucky, and she wondered which of the skills she had learned there would be needed before she and the others were safe again in Allied territory.

As she closed her eyes, she hoped that the gift of easy sleep would prove as much an ally behind enemy lines as it had been all her life. She crunched into the small space between Lois Watson and Richard Lebo and rested her head on her arm to keep her face off the dirty floor. In less than a minute she decided to detach the hood from her raincoat and spread it out as a layer between herself and whatever might be living in the dirt and dust covering the crude floorboards. In the dim light she could see Hassan still sitting upright by the large stone fireplace. His mustached silhouette remained in her mind as she fell asleep.

Suddenly she awakened to the sound of a man's voice, and for several seconds she could not remember where she was. She propped herself on one elbow and tried to determine what had awakened her. The room was filled with the sounds of sleep, the regular breathing of thirty-four people crowded against each other.

Maybe I was dreaming, Jens thought. Everyone seemed to be asleep. Then sounds of mumbling and talking drifted across the room.

That's not a dream, Jens thought. I'm the only one awake, but that's definitely talking. Her mind jumped to a frightening possibility. Had the Germans already tracked them down? Were they outside preparing an assault on this smoke-filled hideout?

The fire had burned very low, making the room darker and colder. Maybe I should awaken Hassan or Lebo, Jens reasoned with herself. Before she could decide, she heard the talking again, louder, across the room—a sleep talker. She resisted the impulse to throw her shoe at the offender. I'd probably miss anyway, she thought. I might as well try to get back to sleep. She turned on her side. The floor felt harder, and for the first time in recent memory, sleep eluded her.

Events from the previous day cascaded through her mind, washed away all hope of sleep, and left a bone-tired weariness in its place. Jens discovered that she was lying in a direct draft coming from beneath the room's ill-fitting outside door. In addition, an icy wind made its way constantly upward through the cracks in the floor. Unsolicited memories of her six weeks' training as a flight nurse at Bowman Field pushed the cold from her mind. For a few brief moments she was in Kentucky again, marching and hiking under an unmerciful August sun, with sweat rolling down her nose and back. Who would have guessed I'd ever miss that heat, she thought, as another gust of wind brought her back to cold reality.

In the dim light of the dying fire she could make out the silhouette of several pieces of wood laying near the wall. Jens got slowly to her hands and knees and stretched herself across a mass of sleep-drenched bodies toward the wood. She managed to pick up a medium-sized chunk and move it slowly back across members of her party, then toss it into the fireplace. She knew it would add to the smoke, but was willing to make that exchange for a little more heat. There was a bright explosion of light as the fuel caught quickly. She looked at her watch. It was 0130.

The luminous dial of her army-issue watch reminded Jens that she did not need firelight to check on the time. I wonder, Jens thought, if they had places like this in mind when they decided what kind of watches air evacuation teams needed to carry. Her mind drifted back to her flight nurse graduation ceremony, and she could feel her uniform soaked with sweat and sticking to her body as her class marched in review in the heat and humidity of a Kentucky summer. Actually, she reflected, this isn't too bad for a night behind enemy lines, but how many nights will there be before we're safe in our own territory? Where would the group go from here, and did Hassan really know what to do with thirty stranded Americans in a German-occupied country? Jens remembered an article she had read in *Reader's Digest* only a month or so ago, the story of an American pilot who had bailed out over German territory and was subsequently hidden and led to safety by partisans. The article spoke of partisans in all enemy territory, partisans who would risk their own lives to aid the Allies and keep their downed fliers out of German hands. But it gave only the bare facts and deliberately omitted the methods used to help this American pilot return to safety. Jens wondered if they would have to remain hidden in this small room indefinitely. She was sure she'd feel better if she could believe for certain that Hassan knew where and how to contact Allied forces with word of where they were and could help keep them alive until arrangements were made to get the thirty Americans back to Italy.

In the dim light of the fire, and lying in the midst of smoke and fellow soldiers, Jens hoped they would be safely back before the military notified their families that they were down and missing in an enemy-occupied country. It was a stroke of good luck that she had gone home on leave in July. Her parents hadn't been happy about her going overseas, and Jens never told them that she had volunteered for duty as a flight nurse. She hadn't been sure how her mom and dad might have reacted to that fact, and she still didn't want to find out.

Jens decided to put another piece of wood on the fire and try again for sleep. The added fuel made a little more warmth as she curled up on the floor again and this time fell almost immediately into sleep.

9 November 1943, Tuesday—0600: Hideout in Albania

Jens and her party were awakened promptly at 0600 by the sleep talker of the previous night. This time he was sitting bolt upright making the announcement, "Okay, kids, show's over!" Jens recognized him as the young corporal from the 802d Squadron who had hitched a ride with them. Corporal Hornsby announced, "I know I talk in my sleep. What did I say?"

"We'll never tell," Pauleen Kanable said. "We'll be listening every night for the continuation of the story." The former American Airlines stewardess from Wisconsin stretched and yawned as she looked at Hornsby, who was pulling on his shoes.

Jens heard someone mention a bathroom and decided she

needed to use it. She got up and stumbled through a low door in the back of the room to find herself in a large bare room that had two tiny windows; it would hardly have qualified as a shed on the farm of Jens's parents back in Michigan. She was shocked to see an old woman asleep on a rough wooden table. The woman didn't stir, and Jens scanned her surroundings for any sign of a bathroom. She spotted a small waist-high partition in one corner and, behind the minuscule screen, a hole cut into the floor of the second-story room. She had to maneuver carefully to avoid stepping into the opening and to keep from scraping her cold, bare buttocks against the crude stone wall of the house. The one-holer was without even the pretense of a toilet seat.

Back in the smoky room, now filled with a dull daylight that filtered through the crooked shutters, some people were sitting up, and others were shaking themselves into wakefulness. It was a disheveled looking crowd of tousle-haired girls, wrinkled uniforms, and the shadow of unshaved stubble on all of the men. Jens made her way back to her sleeping space, stepping gingerly over and between the bodies of her squadron and the plane crew. Her mind and taste buds were longing for hot coffee and a tall glass of fresh orange juice.

There was little conversation since all aspects of the flight had been discussed the previous night. The Americans were encouraged when the owner of the hideout appeared with a pitcher of ice cold water and a basin so they could wash their hands and faces. The man poured the cold water over the hands of each individual, then offered each the same dirty rag to dry them. Everyone was hoping the hand washing meant that food would soon follow, but two hours later food had still not made an appearance.

Jens decided she could use some fresh air. She put on her trench coat and headed for the porch. As she opened the door, she was almost overrun by a group of husky young women, rifles slung across their backs and hand grenades encircling their waists. Each woman was dressed in a dark, coarsely woven, homespun skirt over trousers and wore heavy shoes. Hassan told the Americans that the women had stood guard around the house all night and wanted to greet the Americans personally.

The women partisans attempted to communicate with sign language and a little help from Hassan, but despite high motivation on both sides, conversation did not go well. Undaunted by this setback, these Albanian soldiers decided to sing some of their partisan songs for their visitors—each louder, more fervent, and more rousing than the one before. At the end of every song the women would make a fist and thrust it upward toward the ceiling. Their singing had gotten so loud and raucous that Jens hoped the Germans weren't quite as close as Hassan had said they were. Before leaving, the Albanians shook each American's hand and shouted the Albanian equivalent of "goodbye and good luck." The women tramped heavily out onto the porch and down the flight of rickety wooden steps. Jens wondered how far the news of their arrival had spread.

The sun was peeking through mounds of dark clouds when Jens returned to the porch at 1015 joined by Frances Nelson, Elna Schwant, and Lois Watson. A rainbow that appeared to be several feet wide arched over the side of the mountain and colored the leaves on bushes standing only several paces ahead. The four nurses were joined by a tall, dark sergeant as a cold drizzle began to fall again. No one moved to leave the porch and return to their smoke-filled room.

"About now my roommate is just strolling over to the mess hall for breakfast," Elna said.

"I'll bet Captain Voight and Phillips are each standing on their own airfields scanning the skies for us," Lois said.

"Surely they won't expect us if the weather is as bad as yesterday," Fran said. "Chances are, they don't even know we're missing."

"Our headquarters always sends a message to the docs in Italy that we've taken off," the tall sergeant said. "That is, if they get through on the wireless."

"Do you think we still might fall into German hands even after getting away from the plane safely?" Fran asked.

He shrugged. "It all depends on whether these partisans can keep us hidden and the anti-partisans can be avoided or bought off, and whether the Germans launch an all-out effort to capture us or Hassan and his people can contact someone who can get us out of Albania and back to Italy."

"I don't think they'd mistreat us as prisoners of war, do you?"

"I don't think so," the sergeant said. "You can never be sure about the Krauts."

"I'd hate being confined for the rest of the war," Jens said. "I'd like it even less if we were captured and sent to Germany. The way our boys are bombing German cities in 500- to 800-plane air raids wouldn't make me feel real good about being on the ground there." She pushed the thought out of her mind and deliberately changed the subject. "Besides, I haven't finished addressing my V-mail Christmas cards, and I plan to be back in Sicily very soon."

An Albanian Jens felt sure she hadn't seen before walked onto the porch. He was a slim, middle-aged man with a well-trimmed mustache and a neat, almost western-style suit. He pointed at the English-Italian dictionary in which Jens was writing the beginnings of a diary and started to speak Italian. Jens put up her hands and said, "No compri Italiano." She and the man started looking through the book, and she asked him how to say various Albanian words by pointing to the Italian. She looked at the man and asked, "In what part of Albania are we?"

He took her pen and drew a map of the country on a blank page in the back of the dictionary. He wrote in the towns of Elbasan and Berat, then drew a picture of their plane on the spot where it had landed. Jens looked at the map. They were somewhere in south-central Albania, between the two towns but closer to Elbasan.

Elna interrupted by raising her hand and asking, "Do you hear what I hear? Do you hear? I think it's a plane!"

The sound grew louder and lower. Jens and her companions rushed into the house. "Plane!" Jens shouted. She headed for the back room where she remembered that there were two small windows. The pilots jumped to their feet and followed. Through the low clouds, she caught a glimpse of a single-engine plane.

"It had to be a German, C.B.," Baggs said.

"What kind of plane is a German CB?" Jens asked.

Both pilots laughed.

"I was calling Thrasher by his initials, C.B., for Charles B.," Baggs explained.

"Oh," Jens said. "My one-track mind is on planes."

Thrasher looked at Baggs. "They could be checking this place out for activity, or looking for our plane. What do you think?"

"He didn't circle the house or the area." Baggs sounded relieved.

The German plane headed in the direction of their mired-in transport. Everyone rushed to the porch and watched as it reached the area of their crash landing. The plane didn't circle the site, but everyone agreed that its pilot would have to be either lost or just plain crazy to be flying over this mountainous terrain in such bad weather without some reason.

Throughout the morning, curious neighbors, all men, dropped by to sit by the fire and stare at the Americans. Finally they'd say a few words to the owner of the house or to Hassan, and then leave. Jens couldn't remember seeing any other building nearby and wondered where these people had come from. If secrecy is our ace in the hole, she thought, I'm afraid our celebrity may be our downfall.

As the afternoon wore on, the steady stream of visitors continued. A few men arrived on horseback and spoke with Hassan without dismounting, then quickly turned and rode off.

From several three-way conversations between Hassan and the pilots, Jens surmised that the men on horseback were partisan officials who were giving Hassan instructions on what steps to take next.

She listened with interest as Hassan tried to sell the pilots on his plan to take C.B. to Elbasan to meet the SAS British general, who, he claimed, was in that town. Hassan was certain that he could take Thrasher right to the general with only a minimum of danger.

"We wait few days for your hair," Hassan said, patting his own two-week-old beard, "then dress you like Albanian. You walk with many Albanians, no one think anything. No one talk to you."

Jens readily understood why Hassan asked Thrasher's participation rather than Baggs. Thrasher was of average height and build, had dark hair and brown eyes. Baggs, however, was light complexioned, had reddish blond hair and blue eyes.

Hassan's plan was dropped in a matter of hours. Jens wasn't sure what had killed the idea; she decided that either Hassan was put off by Thrasher's reluctance or the plan had been vetoed by higher partisan leaders.

1600 Hours

The sounds of a scuffle and loud, excited voices in front of the house drew the attention of everyone inside.

Jens and several others peeked out the door to determine what the ruckus was all about. A large black ox was being pushed and pulled toward a tree and was not cooperating one bit. She went out on the porch to get a closer look. To her horror, in a matter of seconds the three men had flipped the ox onto its back and cut its throat. The beast was still kicking as they began skinning and hacking it into pieces. The sight was too much for Jens, and she backed quickly into the house.

"What a gory mess out there!" she said to Thrasher.

Hassan was standing by the fireplace. "Maybe we eat tonight," he said.

"That?" she asked as she pointed over her shoulder.

"Hassan told a partisan official that we'd had nothing to eat since our arrival, so I guess that's supper," Thrasher said.

"Yeah, well, I don't think I could eat a bite of that poor animal," Jens said.

Four hours later, however, when hunks of boiled meat were served on a big tray, Jens ate with relish. The ox was tough and stringy, but no one passed it up as the tray went around.

"Some mashed potatoes would taste good right now," a young sergeant said. "I'd bet this meat could have made pretty good gravy."

"What do you think this is, a standing rib roast?" another man asked between concentrated chewing efforts.

"This stuff could stand without a rib," Lebo said.

"That's what it was doing several hours ago," Jens said.

"What?" Lebo asked.

"Standing!" Jens answered.

"Stop talking about it," Fran said. "I'm trying not to think about it."

The front door flew open, and Baggs, Hassan, and several Albanians walked into the room. They stood for a moment, staring into the firelight.

"Have some supper," Gertrude "Tooie" Dawson passed the tray to them. "It's not exactly like a home-cooked meal in Pittsburgh, but it's better than nothing."

"Where have you been?" Lois asked, still chewing laboriously. "You must be starved."

"I am," Baggs said. He pulled his cap off and took a piece of meat. He lay down by the fire and looked at the meat through half-closed eyes. Jens felt sure he was falling asleep, but then he started to eat, gave a little laugh, and began to tell his comrades of the trouble he'd had setting their plane on fire. He turned toward Thrasher. "I emptied some of the gas out of the wing tank into a container and poured it around inside the plane. My next problem was to find something larger than a kitchen match to fire it. I used the flare gun and shot it through the door. I thought it would take off right away, but after three flares with no success I stepped closer to the door, and when I fired the fourth flare, it caught with a bang. Before I could get my feet into motion in the mud, the explosion caught me and threw me face down in the dirt. My God, what a helpless feeling that was!" He turned toward the radio operator.

"Lebo, do you remember those guys saying they could take the radio out for us without any problem? Well they did, with axes! If it wasn't useless before, it is now!"

"Yeah, I know," Lebo said. "They brought it here about an hour ago."

For the next hour there was little conversation. Suddenly Hassan spoke as if he were telling them the course of their destiny.

"Tomorrow, I take you to Berat, where we get help for you."

"Berat? Where's that?" one of the sergeants asked. "Are there British in Berat?"

Hassan put up his hand and quietly started to explain. "We leave in morning," he said. "Everything is maybe prepared."

"How do we go?" Tooie asked.

"We walk, of course. There is only a trail from here. Very nice trail, but first we check. Some days Germani have, some days, we have."

The group waited for Hassan to continue, but he seemed to have explained everything to his own satisfaction.

"Is Berat a city or a village?" Jean Rutkowski asked. She was sitting cross-legged and putting her short brown hair up in pin curls.

"A very nice city." Hassan sounded proud. "There perhaps we get help for you, and get message to your friends."

The Americans exchanged glances of relief, reassured by the idea that Hassan's people could actually contact the Allies.

"Is it possible to leave early in the morning and get there before dark?" Jens asked.

Hassan ignored her question and continued on his own agenda. "The donkeys won't be here until nine. And before we start, arrangements must be made."

Sergeant Allen expressed the apprehension of many in the group. "I hope the Krauts can arrange to let us have the trail for the day!"

3 Which Way Is Home?

10 November 1943, Wednesday—0850: Hideout

It was almost time for the donkeys to arrive when the nurses scrambled down the outside steps to join the group already waiting on the ground. Jens spotted Baggs and Hassan to the right of the crowd and walked in their direction. She had already decided that she could learn a lot by listening to the talk around her.

Baggs and Hassan appeared deeply involved in their own conversation. Jens stopped near three other nurses and listened. She had to strain a little to hear but was convinced it was worth it.

"How safe will the women be on this journey? How do we know your men won't decide to abuse them?" Baggs asked. His face seemed carved out of stone, and there was no hint of a smile in his eyes. "How do we know all your people will obey you?"

"I tell them already, no touch nurses," Hassan said. "No worry about my people."

"Have you ever had any of them change their minds on the trail? How do you know they'll obey you?"

Hassan narrowed his eyes and flashed his white toothy smile. "They do what I say, or I shoot them!"

Baggs smiled and shook his head. "That's good enough for me. You're a good man, Hassan."

"I good friend to America. If I say I do something, I do it,"

Hassan said in a pleased tone. He pointed down the trail. "The donkeys come. We get ready to go."

"Right," said Baggs.

Jens turned and saw four small donkeys clomping their way to the house. Several Albanians grabbed the nurses' musette bags and secured them on the backs of three of the beasts. Although the crew chief had reported that his knee had improved, the nurses had decided it was better for him to ride than walk, so three medics strapped Sergeant Shumway to the fourth donkey. In less than ten minutes the party was ready to travel.

Hassan mounted his white horse and called for the group to follow him. They pulled off single file along a low stone wall. One of the four Albanian men accompanying the trekkers led Sergeant Shumway's donkey. The other three animals were chased, prodded, and steered by their tails.

The muddy trail was narrow, rocky, and very slick from recent rains. The hikers continued to walk in single file, speaking only to the persons directly ahead and directly behind. After an hour and a half they stopped for a short rest, most sitting down on large rocks.

"What I wouldn't give for a lounge chair," Lillian "Tassy" Tacina said in her characteristically tremulous voice.

"I'd be happy with a kitchen stool," Lois Watson said. "Anything that would let my feet hang down while I rested. I didn't realize it could be so tiring to have my knees up under my chin all the time. I guess I've gotten pretty soft since that tough training at Bowman Field."

"I'll bet that drill-happy lieutenant would love to see us now," Jens said. "Too bad he's not here so we could see how *he* operates in a real emergency situation. This is already worse than those ten-mile hikes at Bowman."

In twenty minutes they were on the trail again. The thick mud sucked the rubber galoshes right off their shoes every nine or ten steps. Jens pulled some two-inch bandage from her medical kit and tied the rubbers to her shoes, then tucked the muddy bottoms of her slacks inside her socks before they continued on the slippery path.

After another hour two squat, crudely built stone houses loomed ahead of them. Within the next thirty minutes, they were led through a gate in a low stone wall and into an enclosed yard. The door of the house was held open by a short, swarthy man who nodded a greeting and beckoned the party to enter. The nurses leaned down and pulled off their galoshes, while the men scraped their muddy GI shoes on the stone steps. As they entered the house, a rustling sound caught their attention. Several Albanian women, shawls on their heads, were sneaking glimpses at the Americans from an adjoining room. The women giggled a few times, then disappeared from sight.

The room was much larger than the one they had shared at the hideout. Two glass windows at eye level allowed light to enter and gave the room a bright appearance. The man of the house motioned for them to sit down on the floor. He reached up and removed two short-legged, handmade tables from hooks on the wall and placed them on the floor in front of the Americans. Nurses and GIs gathered around, two deep. Soon a bowl of hot food was placed on each table, along with several tiny spoons and tin plates with large chunks of cornbread. The group needed no urging to begin digging into the bowls, though it was probably slimmer pickings for those in the outer rows. The large bowls contained steaming rice with chunks of chicken—certainly the best food they had tasted since leaving Catania Main.

It was obvious to Jens that the meal must be part of the arrangements Hassan had spoken of the night before. The food had arrived quickly and in large enough quantities for more than thirty people. I'd bet this is the first time a group of thirty has had to be hidden, fed, and led to safety, Jens thought. Compared to us, one or two pilots to lead out must have seemed like child's play for Hassan and his people. How many Americans would have relished the thought of thirty uninvited and unexpected guests dropping in on them? What single family could house and feed such a crowd? Hassan's arrangements, up to and including this meal, seemed well thought out. She hoped all future arrangements would go as well. She realized that a thousand and one things could interfere with their escape—not the least, the Germans.

As the trekkers dressed to leave, they realized that two galoshes were missing—one of Rutkowski's, and one belonging to Ann Kopsco. They looked everywhere. Hassan questioned the guides, and very explosive conversations ensued, but an hour later the group was back on the trail, minus the galoshes.

The next part of the trail was relatively flat, with many scraggly bushes and an occasional tree. There was less and less conversation as the day wore on; each individual seemed consumed in his or her own thoughts. The simple act of putting one foot in front of the other in the stone-filled mud was a chore that became nature's hostile challenge.

As the group approached a broad river, Jens looked from side to side for the bridge she hoped would be there. At the water's edge it was all too clear that there was no bridge. Then she saw Shumway's donkey being driven across. Two of the other donkeys were standing a foot from the river bank, and two nurses were being loaded on each small animal for the crossing. The guides removed their sandals and rolled their tight pants up above their knees before they waded in, leading the donkeys. The water was only knee deep but moving very fast. Observing the shivering of the guides, Jens concluded that the water was very cold. On successive trips, the donkeys carried the remaining nurses across the rushing current. The medical technicians and plane's crew stripped off their shoes and socks and waded across the icy barrier.

On the other side the trail narrowed and grew steeper. Occasionally some of the Albanian men she had seen when they started out appeared out of the bushes ahead of or behind them, unannounced. Excited verbal exchanges took place between them and Hassan before the men disappeared as quickly as they had appeared. They were obviously scouts, keeping an eye on the trail, and Jens tried to determine from their tone of voice and facial expressions whether the news was good or bad. Hassan's words about Germans using the trail were still strong in her mind.

After two and a half hours they spotted four houses and were ushered quickly into one of them, where they were served rice and cornbread. They tried to heat water in their mess kit cups, hoping to make coffee with the few packets of Nescafe in the meager rations removed from the plane. The handles on the mess cups were too short for the job and conducted heat all too effectively. After several burns, they gave up the idea of instant coffee.

Thoroughly tired out, the group gathered around the fire, talking to stay awake. There were lots of questions for Hassan. The Americans discovered that Hassan had learned to speak English ten years earlier at the Albanian-American school run by the Red Cross. He had gained a lot of skill in his only year at the school and kept in practice by talking to trees, bushes, and frequently to himself. He had left his little village when he joined the partisans in 1939 to fight the invading Italians. He had not been back, and no one in his family knew where he was or what exactly he had been assigned to do.

"But where do the partisans get money to carry on their operations?" Jean asked.

Hassan had a twinkle in his eyes as he said, "From my friend the banker in Tiranë, our capital."

The Americans felt renewed hope when they heard of Hassan's connection. Then he went on to explain that in the early days of the war, the banker would travel to Tiranë occasionally to pick up money for the bank. Hassan and his people would lie in wait for the banker on his return trip. They would go out on the road when they saw his car and demand to know what was in a black box which was used to transport the cash. The banker would answer, "Money," and Hassan would relieve him of that valuable container.

"Now with Germani in country, Albania money is no good," Hassan said.

Jens wondered if Hassan actually had been a bank robber before he joined the partisans.

The sun set and they talked on for several hours. Finally, one by one, the weary army personnel lay down on the hard floor and fell asleep.

11 November 1943, Thursday—0815: On the Trail to Berat

After a breakfast of cornbread the Americans loaded the donkeys and set off for Berat again. The terrain was much the same as the day before, and guides and scouts continued to disappear and reappear in bushes as they hiked. Around 1300 they stopped at a house for a quick lunch of rice and cornbread, then continued up the trail.

Late in the afternoon all the scouts suddenly appeared, stopped the party dead still on the path, and talked in low voices to Hassan. Finally Hassan walked ahead of the Americans, motioned with his finger for quiet, and gestured for them to duck down, saying, "Run fast!"

Each member of the party bent low, and they ran one by one across a barren area. As Jens crossed the clearing she looked to the right to see what she was supposed to be hiding from. They were high on a ridge, and the open area revealed a wide valley far below where she could clearly spot installations, a small hanger, a few small planes, and a short runway. It had to be German but was so far away—at least a mile—they couldn't possibly have been heard. When she asked Hassan about it later, he said, "Yes, but guards up to the top of the mountain sometimes, so we must always be careful!"

The Americans were exhausted that evening when they reached a place called Pashtrani, consisting of four small houses. This time the group spread out among the houses to be more comfortable. They ate chicken and rice again and were feeling the security that three meals a day can give.

Most of the group had taken their shoes and socks off to examine their already sore feet. "This is worse than any trail I've hiked in Utah," said Helen Porter as she draped her damp socks across her shoes.

Only Hassan had enough energy to continue the conversation. The day and the hike seemed routine to him, but the Americans could barely keep their eyes open. Jens tried very hard to stay awake and pay attention to Hassan's stories. She concluded from his words that the partisans felt the Albanian people had an obligation to feed them and, when necessary, to provide them with shelter. Hassan had had many close calls but had never been captured.

"If I captured," Hassan said, "then I be dead."

Jens lay back with the intention of listening to Hassan. The floor was hard and cold. Hiking had made her acutely aware of every muscle and bone in her body. Her feet ached. In less than two minutes, she was sound asleep.

12 November 1943, Friday—0800:
The Trail to Berat

After a breakfast of dry cornbread the nurses stood outside the small stone house, waiting for the men who had slept in the other three houses. At 0815 the party was assembled and on its way again to Berat.

The morning was crisp and filled with sunshine. There had been no rain in the past two days, and the ground was now firm and dry and relatively level. Hassan assured the group that they would be in Berat by noon, or a little sooner. The news lifted their spirits, and conversations were frequent and light as they moved along in single file.

In less than an hour they made their way down a winding trail that took them through a pass and into a wide, sandy valley that had once been a river bed. Helen Porter was riding a donkey, and Jens was playing donkey chaser as she walked alongside. Helen, a native of Utah, was tall and had long brown hair that she had arranged in two braids wrapped around her head—only to find that her uniform cap didn't fit very well. Sitting on that little donkey, cap perched on high, her feet almost dragged the ground.

Suddenly Jens stopped dead in her tracks, focusing all her energy on listening to what she felt sure was a familiar sound. Airplanes, she told herself. Were they from the German airfield they had passed the day before? The sound faded quickly and she began to walk again. The sound returned, only louder. "Listen! Listen!" Jens cried. She looked at the sky expecting to see it darken with hoards of German planes.

Everyone was looking skyward, scanning for the messengers of death—praying that the messages would not fall on them.

The donkeys kept moving, and Jens followed, holding the donkey's tail and looking up at the cloudless sky for planes. The little brown beasts would stop suddenly at unexpected moments to munch and nibble sparse weeds. With each unpredictable stop, Jens walked into the hindquarters of Helen's donkey.

Finally they spotted the planes—and so did the Germans. Guns from all the surrounding hills started barking, and the valley filled to bursting with the sounds of planes and gunfire.

"They're our B-25s; they're ours!" two of the nurses shouted. There were about twelve to fifteen B-25 bombers escorted by eight P-38 fighters. Everyone watched and counted the planes, oblivious to the gunfire shooting skyward from all over the valley's rim.

Suddenly it dawned on the party to take cover, but there was little to conceal them. Helen jumped off the donkey, and she and Jens hid under a nearby scraggly tree. They watched the planes as they flew on toward the next mountain. The guns in the nearby hills let up, and those farther down the valley took over.

"My gosh!" Jens exclaimed. "We've been walking in a valley where the hills are full of guns and Germans. They must have telescopes too—do you suppose they've been watching us prance along here for the past half-hour or more?"

Suddenly there were the sounds of several explosions, and black puffs of smoke filled the air in the far distance.

"We must have hit their fuel supply," one of the medical sergeants said.

The planes soon returned; they didn't fly directly over the valley, but the guns in their area picked up the targets again, in a thunderous roar. One of the bombers was limping far behind. They watched it closely, wondering if they would have more company, but they did not see anyone bail out.

Jens kept her eyes on the planes long after they were just specks in the sky. They reminded her that home was out there someplace, and she must continue moving toward it.

In half an hour Berat lay ahead of them, and Jens hoped that this city would provide the help they needed to return to their own lines—to the military home they had left in Sicily four days earlier.

4 Germans Attack

12 November 1943, Friday—1230: Berat

They entered the town of Berat on a cobblestone street lined with people who had come out to greet them. The crowd sang songs, threw flowers at the Americans' feet, and snapped their pictures. The group was flabbergasted. How did these people know they were coming? How did they know their time of arrival? Jens felt a mixture of appreciation and apprehension. How could their movements and whereabouts be secret when so many people knew the answers to both questions?

The party was led through the town to the steps of the schoolhouse, where city officials greeted them and gave speeches to celebrate their arrival. One man translated the speeches in better-than-average English. Jens could scarcely believe her ears. According to the translator, the Albanians were welcoming them as an invasion force who had finally come to help them. How could anyone mistake a group of seventeen men and thirteen women, all limping from the red areas on their heels, for an invasion force? She looked at Ann Maness who, like herself, had used two-inch bandage across her head and tied beneath her chin in order to hold her uniform cap on in the strong, cold wind that never seemed to stop. Quite an army!

Before she could answer her own questions or sort out her thoughts, they were led to a small hotel for a lunch of cold mutton, rice, and cornbread. Afterward, they were paraded up and down the main street, then led to a small hall where a large contingent of people greeted them. In less than an hour the Americans were assigned in twos and threes to spend the night in individual homes.

Jens was delighted when she and Wilma Lytle, a native of Kentucky, were assigned to the home of the translator. It was certainly a plus to be housed where someone spoke English. The man introduced himself as Kostig Steffa.

It was almost sundown when they arrived at Steffa's comfortable two-story home. They followed their host through a long hall, past a room lined with straight chairs, to the top of a narrow stairway and into a cozy living-dining room combination. The room was heated by a potbellied stove that provided uniform warmth without the smoke produced by the fireplaces.

Steffa introduced his wife and elderly parents, then asked Jens and Wilma to make themselves comfortable. Mrs. Steffa, a slim, dark-haired woman who spoke minimal English, taught elementary school in Berat. The couple had five children, the youngest three months old.

"Your English is so good," Jens said to their host. "I can't help but wonder if you attended school outside of Albania."

Steffa smiled. "Yes, I went to school in Italy a few years but have never been in an English-speaking country."

Like Hassan, he had learned English at the Albanian-American school. Unlike Hassan, Steffa had spent four years there.

"Did you know Hassan when you attended that school?" Jens asked.

"No. I'm sure he is a younger man. He most likely attended after I had finished there," Steffa said. "Mr. Fultz was the headmaster and taught us much about your country and its history."

"I hope you don't mind my asking," Jens said, "but I'm curious as to why your people thought we were an invasion force."

"My people have waited a long time for America to send us help so we could fight more effectively against the Germani. When the word spread of your arrival, people thought the American invasion had started."

"But with thirteen women, how could they think we were the beginning of an invasion force?" Jens asked.

"Our women are guerrillas and have fought along with our men for years," Steffa said.

"I hadn't thought of that," Wilma said. "Actually we met some of your women who guarded us the first night we were here. They came in the next morning and sang partisan songs for us."

"My people have always looked up to your country for its stand on democracy," Steffa said. "We even have a city named Port Wilson in honor of one of your presidents."

"Was there a special reason you chose President Wilson?" Wilma asked.

"He was the only person who spoke for Albania in the League of Nations when it seemed likely our country would be divided between Greece and Yugoslavia after World War I. We felt he understood even a small country's desire for freedom." He leaned forward. "If you and the British would arm us, we could do a lot more to fight the Germans. We have begged and begged for arms and equipment, yet they never come."

Jens wasn't sure what to say. It seemed ironic that a people she had heard so little about in world history now stood between her and capture or even death at the hands of the Nazis. Steffa and his countrymen had to know next to nothing about the political influence of a second lieutenant in the Army Nurse Corps.

Steffa's political conversation slowed during supper. His wife asked questions about life in the Army Nurse Corps, and his mother seemed intent upon every word. Steffa alternated his attention between translating for his parents and giving directions in Italian to the houseboy who was serving the meal. Jens remembered what Hassan had told her of the many Italian soldiers who had been stranded in Albania when Italy signed a truce with the Allies in September.

Jens was beginning to feel the activities of the last three days. "I'm afraid I'm going to have to excuse myself," she said. "I'm what we Americans refer to as 'bone-tired.'"

But as Jens and Wilma stood up, they became keenly aware that Steffa's mother was sitting with a very worn deck of cards, waiting for her turn to socialize with the Americans. They moved over to another table and played a few spirited games of what turned out to be fan-tan. His mother was extremely pleased that the American women knew her favorite card game.

Jens and Wilma slept in the house next door. It had belonged to the mayor, but he had left some time ago, for political reasons. The nurses were given the mayor's bedroom.

"A bed!" they exclaimed as they entered the room. Jens planned to stay awake long enough to roll around in the bed a few times before she went to sleep. She lay down on the bed and slept until morning.

13 November 1943, Saturday—0900: Berat

There was a knock at the door at 0900. Jens opened the door to be greeted by a small boy who bowed to the women. He was the Steffas' ten-year-old, Alfredo, who had come to lead them back to his parents' house. Hot tea was served, but it was chamomile tea. The leaves grew in the mountains, they were told. Neither woman cared for chamomile tea, but a cup of anything hot tasted good at that moment. It went well with the toasted cornbread and a very strong, white cheese that Steffa said was made from goat's milk. After breakfast, he explained that plans had been made to take the group to see a shrine and to meet more of the townspeople.

Small versions of army trucks picked up all thirty of them, plus a few Albanians. They were so crowded that most of the group had to stand. They bumped their way down the only street in Berat capable of supporting vehicle traffic and entered a cemetery, where they were led to the tall monument of a fallen Albanian hero; then it was back again to be shown one of the town's two schools. They walked along the main street but saw no evidence of shops of any kind that were still in business. Jens was amazed that their hosts wanted to show them about rather than keep them indoors until contacts had been made and arrangements completed to spirit them out of the country. She was eager to ask the pilots whether they had made any contacts or found any facilities for sending messages, but they were surrounded by officials attended by Steffa as interpreter.

The group was taken again to the hotel for lunch. Jens wondered who was picking up the bill for such a large party. Food wasn't what could be called abundant, and American money wasn't any good in Albania.

Hassan came around the long table to say goodbye to each American individually. He was leaving to return to his area. Jens and the party had become fond of him in the last few days and thanked him for his help this far.

After lunch they were taken to an upstairs meeting hall where quite a few Albanian men were already gathered. As they were introduced, Jens realized that most of them were city officials, and to her consternation the speeches started all over again.

13 November 1943, Saturday—1330: 61st Troop Carrier Squadron, Army Air Forces, Office of the Operations Officer

A missing aircraft report and memorandum were issued on 13 November 1943. The memo, directed to "Commanding Officer, 314th Troop Carrier Group, OAF, APO 760. US Army," follows:

1. On November 8th at 0900, Army Aircraft 42-68809, a C-53D left Catania with Bari, Italy as its destination. It was carrying twenty five [twenty-six] (26) passengers besides its crew of four. These people are listed below.
2. It has been learned that radio contact was established between the plane and the station at Bari. The first contact was made at 1031. At this time the Pilot asked for the weather at Bari. The station challenged him but he was unable to answer the challenge so they did not give out the information desired. At 1050 contact was made again and the Pilot asked that the beacon be turned on. He was again unable to answer the challenge and the beacon was not turned on. At 1120 he asked for the beacon again with no results. At 1135 he asked to be given a radio fix but the station was unable to do this as they do not have the necessary equipment. The pilot again asked for the beacon and at 1145 it was turned on for ten minutes although the Pilot was

still unable to identify himself. The radio station was unable to make contact with the plane after this time.

3. One plane was sent from this squadron on November 11th, to search for the missing plane. It covered the area as well as possible but was not able to make a thorough search because of the size of the area involved. All airports in the area were contacted but the plane was not found.

4. We assume that the plane must be either in the mountains on the toe of Italy or in the Gulf of Taranto or the Adriatic Sea or, it is possible that he might have landed in Greece.

5. It is suggested that a thorough search of the area be made.

6. The complete names, rank and serial numbers were not available at the time of the search but can be obtained along with other information regarding the passengers from Major McKnight at Catania. Major McKnight may be reached by phone at Tallyho-48.

Pilot:	Thrasher, Charles B.	1st Lt
Co-pilot:	Baggs, James A.	2nd Lt
Crew Chief:	Shumway, Willis L.	Sgt.
Rad Opr:	Lebo, Richard	Sgt.

Passengers

Nurses	**EM**
2nd Lt Dawson	T/Sgt Abbott
2nd Lt Porter	T/Sgt Adams
2nd Lt Maness	T/Sgt Allen
2nd Lt Markowits [Markowitz]	T/Sgt Cranson
2nd Lt Rutowski	T/Sgt Cruise
2nd Lt Lytla [Lytle]	T/Sgt Eberg
2nd Lt Schwant	T/Sgt Eldridge
2nd Lt Naleson [Nelson]	T/Sgt Hayes
2nd Lt Watson	T/Sgt MacKinnon
2nd Lt Jansen [Jensen]	T/Sgt Owen
2nd Lt Taoina [Tacina]	T/Sgt Wolf
2nd Lt Kopsco	T/Sgt Zaibar [Zeiber]
2nd Lt Kanable	

It was signed "For the Commanding Officer: Gordon E. Hein, 1st Lieutenant, Air Corps."

13 November 1943, Saturday—1645:
Berat

All the speeches had one overriding theme: "Tell the Americans and British to send us arms to fight the Germans. Tell them to send us supplies so we can continue our patriotic battle."

Under the circumstances, about all the pilots could do was thank them over and over for their help and the many kindnesses shown to this group of stranded Americans.

It was late afternoon when they emerged from the hall and once more were parceled out in twos and threes to various waiting people who led them to their homes for the night. Again Jens was lucky enough to be in a home where one person spoke English. The family served Jens and Wilma Lytle a mutton stew for supper. The fat in the stew stuck to the roof of Jens's mouth, but she remembered the days of no food and ate it all. Several hours later the two were served a strong, sweet, syrupy Turkish coffee in a dainty little demitasse cup and saucer.

"Your china is very beautiful," Jens said to their hosts.

"Thank you," their host said. "People have hidden their best dishes and household items. We'd rather hide them than the Germans get hold of them. If the Germans ever decide to take Berat, they'd loot every house for food, fuel, and anything else they might use or want." The host cleared his throat. "Of course, that's not the worst of it. The Germans have looted scores of villages and towns, and they always take ten or twenty hostages. In a town this size every hostage is a friend or relative of someone in town. The Germans tell us, 'If you don't cooperate, the hostages will never be returned.' The first hostages taken two years ago have never come back, and no one knows what happened to them." He shook his head. "That's why we have no faith in the word of Germans."

Jens thought that this stocky, middle-aged man must be a lawyer, but she couldn't decide whether he worked for the government or practiced privately. The man gave no evidence that he might be willing to discuss his profession.

Jens and Wilma were pleasantly surprised to learn that they had a bedroom and a fluffy feather mattress for the night. Their hostess apologized, with her few English words and many gestures, for not having an extra blanket to offer them, but shrugged as she indicated that an extra blanket would only keep some German warm if they decided to take their town.

14 November 1943, Sunday—0900:
Berat

Officials took the Americans to the town hall for more political meetings, once again stressing the urgent need of Albanians for arms and other supplies from America. Jens could scarcely believe her eyes when the officials followed their speeches with movies addressing the political situation in Albania. A late lunch at the home of a prosperous partisan topped off a sunny Sunday afternoon.

Jens was glad the party was again broken into twos and threes and assigned to various homes for the night. She and Ann Kopsco arrived at their assigned home in time for cornbread, cheese, and tea. They were happy to be shown to their bedroom immediately after their meal, as no one in the house spoke a word of English. They were surprised that the bed sagged almost to the floor when they climbed into it. There were covers, however, and Jens and Ann were able to get undressed for sleep.

15 November 1943, Monday—0715:
Berat

It was barely daylight when a loud boom awakened the women. It sounded like thunder, but as Jens listened more carefully to the boom! boom! boom! there was no mistaking the sound. It was heavy gunfire. Jens turned and looked at Ann, whose huge brown eyes seemed even larger in her small face. There were two more booms before they struggled out of that low, sagging bed and crawled on hands and knees to peer out of the tiny windows. All they could see were rooftops. The town seemed perfectly calm in the early morning light, but they could hear the guns, unmistakable now, in an almost continuous barrage. They grabbed their slacks and shirts, stepped into their shoes and headed for the front door where their host was already standing, clasping and unclasping his hands and looking as if he had seen a legion of ghosts. Jens nodded to the man and his wife as she ran past them to get out on the front steps. While they were trying to determine where the roar of guns was coming from and which way they should go, a couple of sergeants came running down the road in front of the house.

"Hey!" both women shouted. "What is all the noise about, and where are you going?"

"Darned if we know, but we're going to the hotel to find out what the pilots want to do."

"Are you coming back?" Jens yelled.

"Yeah, we have to come back to get our gear," one sergeant called back.

"Well, let us know what the word is, will you?" Jens called out after them and rushed back to their bedroom to finish dressing and to pick up their few belongings.

The loud booming continued in sporadic bursts. As the two nurses made a dash for the door again, their hosts pointed at a table set for breakfast.

"No, no, thank you," the nurses said. They shook hands hurriedly and got to the porch in time to catch the out-of-breath sergeants running uphill and hear them shout.

"The pilots want everyone at the hotel."

Jens and Kopsco took off at a trot. The hotel and only road through town were at the foot of the hill. Thrasher and Baggs were standing on the front steps of the hotel, where the crew and several nurses had spent the night. As Jens and Ann got closer, the pilots yelled at them, "Go on out that road. Just follow the crowd. Some of the others are ahead of you. We'll catch up to you as soon as we get a truck."

"Okay," Jens called back. Both nurses waved as they were virtually swept along with the crowd. The only street in Berat was full of people who were moving like a human tide, through and out of the town. Some carried possessions; some rode in horse-drawn carts; but all moved with one will—to escape Berat.

The gunfire had stopped as abruptly as it had begun. Jens and Ann hurried to catch up with two sergeants they could see far ahead.

Each time Jens looked at Ann, those big eyes seemed to get

larger. "I can't believe I brought these shoes instead of my GI boots," Ann said. "I have a feeling these thin soles and slightly higher heels will be a problem before we see Italy again."

Jens could make out Tassy, Marky, and Sergeant Owen in the crowd ahead. The sergeant was riding a large brown horse in the field that ran alongside the road. Try as she might, Jens could not distinguish any individual among the hordes of Albanians.

They hadn't traveled far when a bright orange truck carrying the pilots and about a dozen of their party came racing up behind them. Several hands reached down to haul Jens and Ann and others of their party on board. So many Albanians climbed on as well that there was soon standing room only.

Jens tried to look over the crowd and count heads for their group. "Have you seen Nelson, Watson, or Schwant?" she called to the Americans.

"Yes," one of the nurses responded. "I saw Watson and Nelson anyway. They must be on ahead."

Suddenly Jens recognized Sergeant Zeiber, who had run downhill by their house along with Sergeant Abbott, and then she identified Steffa, seated with his back against the cab of the truck. He looked dazed and frightened, and merely nodded in her direction without a word. Jens could hardly believe that this frightened, preoccupied refugee was the vibrant leader she had known only days before. How could this be? Surely Steffa and the other officials were no strangers to the murderous whims of the Nazis.

The truck stopped with a jerk, and several more of the party, all men, were pulled on board.

"Have you seen any others in our group this morning?" Jens asked the new arrivals.

"Yeah. We saw Nelson and a couple of the others earlier. They must be ahead of us," a sergeant answered.

"Has anyone seen Maness?" Jens asked. There was silence for several seconds. Finally, Tooie Dawson spoke up. "No. I don't think anyone has seen her since last night."

Jens tried again to count heads but the large number of Albanians standing and squatting on the truck made an accurate tally impossible.

"Are all or most of the men here?" Jens asked Baggs.

He shook his head. "I don't even know half of them by name yet."

They searched the crowds as the truck rumbled and bumped along the rocky road. Without warning three small planes appeared directly overhead, flying low and heading straight for Berat.

"Stukas!" Baggs yelled. The truck stopped abruptly, throwing everyone forward. They exited the truck from all sides, hitting the ground with bone-jarring force. Jens landed feet first in a mud puddle.

"Oh, damn!" she exclaimed.

The planes were well past them before everyone was off the truck. Jens looked in the direction of the town and realized that the loud booming sound had returned with more ferocity than before.

"My God!" Jens exclaimed. "The Germans are bombing Berat!"

The truck driver's voice could be heard above the crowd. He was waving frantically for everyone to get back on the truck. The loading process took more than five minutes since most had to be pulled up. They had ridden only a few hundred feet when three more planes flew overhead. The riders leaped from the truck again, taking cover in the sparse plants along the sides of the rough road. Again the Stukas, flying low, headed straight for Berat.

They scrambled aboard the big orange truck again, and again the truck traveled away from the town.

"Did you see Maness?" Jens asked Baggs. "She's tall and has long braids wrapped around her head."

"Yeah, now I know who you mean," Baggs said. "But I haven't seen her today."

"And Porter?" Tassy called to Baggs. "She has long hair in braids too."

Baggs shook his head. "No, I haven't seen her since last night."

"And Lytle? I haven't seen her," Fran said. "We haven't picked her up yet either."

"Has anyone seen them?" Jens yelled.

"Who?" one of the sergeants asked.

"Lytle, Maness, and Porter," Fran called again.

The sergeants shook their heads. Sergeant Shumway's voice cut across other conversations.

"Planes!" he yelled. The truck stopped before the word was completely out of his mouth.

The Stukas came over the top of a huge hill that skirted the road. They were already overhead before half of the people were off the truck. As they reassembled minutes later, Baggs yelled, "Let's stay off this bright orange target, and get off the road too." He pointed up the hillside. "Go up there and into the brush until we know the planes have left."

The Americans scrambled up a dry, grassy hill to some high bushes, crawled under them, and lay down. The planes circled and turned, then took another run at Berat.

"They can't carry that many bombs, can they?" Tassy asked Thrasher, who was lying under a nearby bush.

"Naw, they're probably dropping them one at a time to harass the population," Thrasher answered. "After they unload all their bombs, they'll unload their guns at any likely target."

Baggs's voice came from nearby scrub. "That's why I got away from that damn truck. It will be a prime target when they get around to it. They might even spray that road full of refugees if they decide to be real nasty."

The pilots continued discussing the planes and the fuel supply they might have. "They'll probably have to go for more bombs and fuel within the next hour," Thrasher said.

Before Baggs could reply, the sound of low-flying planes filled the air. This time the aircraft stayed behind the hill and out of sight from the Americans' hiding place. Suddenly there was the unmistakable chatter of machine gun fire.

"They must be strafing the road," Tassy said. "Maybe the truck too!" She sounded frightened.

"I wonder if Steffa got back on the truck," Jens said. She looked around to see if he might have joined them under the bushes. Quite a few Albanians had taken cover with their party, but as far as Jens could see, Steffa wasn't with them. In a minute or so the Stukas flew high above them, heading back to their base.

A young Albanian sat nearby, looking at Berat through field

glasses. He chattered excitedly and pointed toward the town. Thrasher and Baggs slid over to him and reached out for the glasses. The boy handed them quickly to Baggs, gesturing wildly with his hands. He stopped abruptly and stared at the pilots.

"What is it? What is it?" the boy asked.

"Tanks or some other vehicles coming into Berat from the other side of town," Baggs said. "Half-tracks! That's what they are— half-tracks." The three watched quietly, passing the glasses back and forth.

"They're not stopping," Baggs said. "They're coming right along Berat's one street."

Thrasher reached for the glasses. "Let me take another look."

In fifteen minutes, even without field glasses the Americans could see German vehicles on the road they had traveled out of town. They were moving fast.

"Don't you suppose they want Berat after that show of force? Was it just to use the road through town, or for some other reason?" Elna asked no one in particular.

"I wonder what's down that road that they're so anxious to reach," Lebo said.

"Maybe they want to head off some of those refugees to question them," Sergeant Adams said.

The group watched Berat for further action or troop movements, but the town seemed totally quiet.

The pilots discussed which way their group should go. It was unanimous that they should head away from Berat, but what about the Germans on the road?

The boy with the binoculars was trying to tell them something, using unrelated English words and hand gestures.

"You speak English?" Baggs asked.

"Very leetle," he said. "My name is Szhanny."

Jens and the group decided the boy was trying to say "Johnny."

Baggs asked the boy if there was a village nearby and off the road, where they might get shelter for the night.

He nodded quickly and pointed over his shoulder, speaking what they thought was probably the name of the town. The group encircled Johnny so they could hear every word he said. His English was poor, but they felt he understood them, and they decided to follow him.

"Come on, come on," Johnny said. "We're leaving."

A quick look told Jens and the others that about half their group was there. They called out all the names they could think of while they spread out and searched for their missing companions. There were no answers to their calls, and when they reassembled, they counted seventeen of their party present.

"Which nurses are missing?" Baggs asked.

"Markowitz, Rutkowski, Kanable, and Dawson," Jens answered, "in addition to the three we couldn't find earlier."

"That means six of our men are also missing," Baggs said. "My God! You don't think they went on with the truck do you?"

Jens's mind was filled with thoughts of the strafing. She wondered how things could get so mixed up on one simple maneuver.

Two of the sergeants started talking about going back into Berat to find Helen Porter, Ann Maness, and Wilma Lytle.

"Does anyone know where they stayed? Were they together?" Jens asked Sergeant Zeiber.

Tassy thought they were together, but no one knew where.

"I should think their 'family' would head them out of town but may have taken them by a different route," Sergeant Adams said. "Surely they don't want Americans in their houses now."

Baggs looked at Sergeant Wolf as he spoke, "I don't think you'd accomplish much by returning to Berat. Surely they left town when the guns started firing. Even if they were delayed for some reason, they must have left Berat by now."

"If those three are still in Berat, or have gone off in some other direction, then ten of our people may have been with the truck," Jens said to herself as much as to anyone else.

Sergeant Lebo was looking through the binoculars. "There are more half-tracks, cars, and trucks entering Berat. Some are coming on through and some are unloading," he said.

"They're right here on the road below us," Tassy said.

"What's the next town from here? Where does that road lead? Why are the Germans moving beyond Berat?" Jens shot the questions at Johnny in rapid-fire succession.

The boy looked at her in bewilderment. His only answer was to urge the group to follow him up the hill. After ten more minutes of discussion the Americans fell into line behind their young guide, but kept looking back, hoping to see members of their group hurrying to catch up.

15 November 1943—1400:
Headquarters, 314th Troop Carrier Group,
Army Air Force, APO 760

Memorandum:
Subject: Missing Air Crew Report
To: Commanding General, 52nd Troop Carrier Wing, Army Air Force, APO 760
1. Transmitted herewith Missing Air Crew Report on aircraft C-53, 42-68809, 61st T.C. Sq., 314th T.C. Gp., on flight from Catania—Cape Collone—Grottaglie—Bari.
2. This aircraft missing in non-battle casualty status.
For the Group Commander:
Richard R. Baker, Jr.
Capt., A.C.
Adj.
Incl.
Missing Air Crew Report (in quin).

15 November 1943, Monday—1700:
Village South of Berat

Several hours after leaving their hiding place outside Berat the Americans arrived at a village comprising three houses. Two Albanian men approached, and Johnny engaged them in lengthy conversation. Jens wondered why it was taking so long.

"What gives, Thrasher?" Jens called to the pilot. "Do you have any idea whether we can stay here?"

Thrasher tapped Johnny on the arm and he stopped long enough for C.B. to ask, "Can we stay here?"

Johnny nodded. "We stay here." He said a few words to the

men, and they led the party into a house without stopping their conversation. When Johnny finally did stop talking for a few minutes, he managed to get across to the group that they could stay in all three houses. A loud protest went up. "No, let's stick together even if we have to sleep in shifts," Tassy said. "If we split up, more of us might get separated."

They huddled together in a tiny, smoky room, even smaller and dingier than the room in the first house, but the warmth of the fire felt great in the increasing coldness as night approached. The party sat silently, too numb or too stunned to carry on a conversation. Occasionally someone shifted position or tossed a piece of wood on to the fire. Finally, Tassy broke the silence.

"I'd still like to know what and why the Germans chased down that road, and whether our gang was on that truck when it was strafed."

"We don't know for sure that the Germans strafed the truck," Sergeant Adams said.

"Do you suppose the Germans knew we were in Berat?" Ann Kopsco asked.

"If they didn't know before, they sure know now. But they didn't have to make all that fuss to get us out of town," Sergeant Lebo said.

"Maybe they didn't expect us to move as fast as we did," Elna said. "Maybe they planned to catch us with their half-tracks."

"It's more likely they were after the road and Berat, and we were in their way," Sergeant Wolf said. "It's almost impossible to figure which way they'll fan out when we don't know their objective."

The group hadn't seen a real road since they left the orange truck, and their efforts to get information from Johnny concerning the nearest road and where it would lead were futile. Suddenly Johnny didn't seem to understand anything. The possibility of being captured by the Germans loomed greater and more real than at any time since their crash landing.

"Remember those survival courses at Bowman Field?" Lois asked. "They told us that if we were captured, all the information we should give the Krauts was our name, rank, and serial number."

"Oh, be quiet, Lois," Fran Nelson said. "Who wants to think about being captured?"

The entire party fell back into stony silence. Jens reached into her pocket for her wallet and went through its contents. Anything with names and addresses on them she tossed into the fire. She looked around the room and saw that the others were doing the same.

"You know what just hit me?" Jens asked.

"What?" Lois asked.

"We should have done this the first night, when we learned we were in enemy territory."

"Gee, that's right," Lois said. "Somehow we tend to be trusting souls, don't we? Or is the word 'stupid'?"

Jens pulled a postcard picture out of her jacket pocket. A photographer in Berat had taken the picture of Ann Maness and Jens when they entered the town. Both women had used two-inch bandage to tie their caps on their heads. They looked a little like Jacob Marley when he visited Scrooge on Christmas Eve. Jens smiled as she looked at the photo. I'd really like to keep it, she thought. "Oh, well!" Jens said aloud, as she turned the photo over to reveal Hassan's name and address. Hassan had written it on the photo himself so the Americans could visit him after the war. Jens hated the thought of burning the photo but knew that if she were captured, the name and address could lead the Germans directly to Hassan and his family. She tossed it into the fire, and as she watched it burn, she wondered where Ann Maness could be.

16 November 1943, Tuesday—0730: On the Trail to Matishave

The next morning two Albanians came into the room, talked with Johnny, and motioned for them to leave the house.

"Where are we going?" Jens asked.

Johnny ignored all questions and continued to gesture that the group should leave quickly. The two men who had talked to Johnny were pacing the small room and letting their worry beads move slowly through their fingers. Worry was the operative word, since with the Germans on the move in the area, they obviously didn't want the

Americans to loiter a minute longer than absolutely necessary. The group had become even more dangerous to any Albanian who dared to give them shelter.

They followed Johnny up a trail, and once they were out of sight of the house, they stopped Johnny and again told him about their missing American friends.

"Does this trail lead to a village where we're likely to find them?" Jens asked.

"Friends?" Johnny said. He looked puzzled. Baggs went over the entire story again, slowly, and with much gesturing. Suddenly, Johnny's eyes lit up. "Ah, ten more!" He nodded thoughtfully. "Yes, come with me."

The Americans felt encouraged and quickly fell into line behind Johnny. Three hundred feet down the path they met a large, motley band of men, many dressed in dilapidated Italian army uniforms. They stepped off the path to let the Americans pass, but when Jens looked back ten minutes later, the entire band—approximately 150 men—was following their group.

Each time they entered a small village, they'd prod Johnny to ask the people about three women who would be dressed in blue uniforms like those the women of the group were wearing, and about the other four women and six men who were missing. As soon as Johnny stopped talking, they encircled him and began asking questions.

"Do they know anything about the other Americans?" someone would ask.

Johnny's quick nod and wave of his hand to indicate that they should follow was all the party needed to rush on behind him.

The Italians and partisans had swelled their ranks to that of a small army. When they took time out to rest at noon, Jens felt more concern than ever. They hadn't met anyone for hours, and she wondered if Johnny really knew where he was leading them. If they were going in the wrong direction, they might never catch up to the rest of their group. Jens was considering the possibilities when an Italian officer appeared before her and introduced himself as a major in the medical corps. In passable English he said he had recognized the caduceus on their uniforms and wondered what American nurses were doing in Albania. Jens related their story and asked if his group had seen any other Americans.

"No," he said. "In fact, I was surprised to see any Americans, since we had heard nothing of an invasion." He went on to explain that he and his people were among a large number of Italians stranded in Albania after their country capitulated to the Allies in September. He wanted information about conditions in Italy, but Jens and her group could tell him little, since they had been in Italy for only a few weeks before their ill-fated flight.

A long sloping hill rose in front of the party. It was sparsely vegetated and had no particular trail. In fact, it was composed mainly of large slabs of slate, set at an angle steep enough to make walking on them all but impossible. The cold drizzle that had fallen earlier made the surface of the slate even slicker. The Americans slipped and slid. In some places it was necessary for them to crawl on their hands and knees over the rocks, acquiring new scrapes and cuts on their kneecaps and trying not to lose more ground than they gained. As they approached the top, scattered patches of dirt made walking somewhat easier, but only for about twenty-five feet. Jens glanced back and realized that the Italians were no longer in sight.

Suddenly a shot rang out, and a bullet whizzed by Jens's head; four more shots followed in rapid succession. Everyone dropped to the ground and froze for a full two minutes. In the silence there wasn't a clue as to who had fired. At last Baggs passed the word to start crawling toward a stone house they could see at the top of the ridge. In a few minutes several people tried to get to their feet, but as soon as they straightened up, two shots rang out. Everyone reverted to crawling, and in fifteen minutes the Americans had reached the house and were huddled against one of its outside walls. One of the sergeants leaned forward to see if he could locate the door. More shots.

"They're damned poor shots," Sergeant Adams said. "They didn't even hit the building." He took off in a crouch with two or three men following him; in moments he called out, "The door is just a few feet this way." Three or four more ran, and only one shot rang out.

"Let's all make a dash for the door before they get us lined up in their sights," Sergeant Zeiber called. "Just make sure you crouch down low and run. The gunfire is coming from the ridge across that narrow valley, so if we stay low, we have a good chance to make it—let's go!"

Everyone followed the sergeant toward the door, and in minutes the entire group was inside the stone house. Its one window, as luck would have it, looked out on the ridge where the shooters were dug in.

"Stay away from the window," Baggs called. "And stay close to the floor."

Jens looked at Johnny. "Germans?" she asked.

He shrugged his shoulders. "Maybe Ballista!"

"Ballista? What are Ballista?" Jens asked. The two had the attention of the group.

"Albanians, not partisans," Johnny said. He gestured with a raised arm salute. "They fight for Germans."

"Oh, great!" Jens exclaimed. "When we don't have the Germans after us, the Ballista are trying to kill us for them." She looked at Johnny again. "How many Ballista are there?"

She might as well have asked for a list of their names, as Johnny seemed to nod and shake his head alternately, no matter what question he was asked.

"Well, however many of them are out there," Baggs said, "they have a lot more gun power than we do at the moment." He held up his submachine gun and tapped the .45 that Thrasher wore in a shoulder holster. Both weapons had been salvaged from the plane before Baggs set it on fire.

The group sat on the dirt floor and leaned against the thick stone wall.

"These walls should stop anything they've got," Sergeant Zeiber said. "As long as we stay clear of that window."

"True," Baggs agreed. "But we have no guards posted. If they got close enough, they could lob a grenade right through the window."

"Not from that ridge over there, they can't," Thrasher said.

"Let's hope all of them stay on that ridge," Sergeant Zeiber said. "It would be a long open dash to a protected area if we needed to get out of here fast."

Suddenly three Albanian men appeared at the door. One, supported by his two comrades, was hopping on one leg. Gunfire rang out, and bullets splattered very near the doorway. The men crouched and fell into the room.

"Put him over here," Jens called.

The two men deposited their friend and disappeared out the door.

The wounded man's pant leg was soaked with blood. Jens ripped the cloth away from the wound and exposed a nasty gash on his thigh, which bled profusely. The man had bitten his lower lip until it too bled; he was obviously in severe pain. Tassy held a pressure bandage on the wound while Jens took a morphine syrette from her medical kit—the first syrette to be used out of a case split up among the nurses—and administered the morphine. They cleaned the wound and dressed it with sulfa powder and a clean bandage. The man had just drifted off into sleep when two more wounded men came hobbling into the room, though neither was hurt as badly as the first man. Jens and Tassy cleaned and dressed their injuries as well.

It was 1400, and an hour had passed without any gunfire from the ridge. Hoping that the people doing the shooting had found more interesting targets, the group decided that they needed to get away before nightfall; the cover of darkness would allow their attackers to close in on the house and kill its current inhabitants. The plan was to run for the cover of a nearby stone wall and then make their way farther up the trail to the next partisan village.

Three sergeants made a trial dash for the wall, but gunfire rang out immediately. Bullets smashed into the dirt around their feet and drove the sergeants back into the house. There was another volley of gunfire, and two more wounded appeared and were cared for by the nurses. Fifteen minutes later a young man walked in and spoke to Johnny. He apparently told him that it was clear for them to leave, since Johnny gestured for the Americans to follow him out of the house. This time they dashed for the low stone wall without a shot being fired at them. As they raced away from the house, darkness closed in, and Jens hoped that Johnny knew where he was leading them.

After five and a half hours of hiking, the party arrived at another village of three houses. Jens looked at her watch; it was 2200, and except for a few barking dogs in the distance everything was quiet. Johnny shook the metal gate of the first house they reached. In less than a minute, a very sleepy looking man appeared at the gate with a gun in his hand. He and Johnny spoke in half whispers and soon the gate was swung open. The man motioned for them to follow him quickly as he ran ahead and opened the door to a small smoke-filled room where people were lying around the fire. They looked at the Americans without an ounce of curiosity, as if the appearance of strangers was not at all unusual. Almost in unison they moved closer to the fire and each other, leaving room for the seventeen Americans and their Albanian guide to join them on the floor. Jens calculated that the space from the firebox to the wall could not have been much over five feet wide. After removing her soggy shoes and socks and inspecting her aching feet, she lay down on the floor and tried to keep her feet out of the fire. She stayed awake only long enough to wonder why she was neither hungry nor thirsty, since she had had no water all day and no food since Sunday in Berat.

5 Separated and Lost

Only ten minutes after awakening, the group questioned Johnny again about the missing members of the party.

"Do these people know anything about the other Americans?" Jens asked.

Johnny looked puzzled. "Other Americans?" he asked.

"Yes, ten others, ten more Americans," Baggs said.

This time they tried more elaborate sign language to try to get their message across: they lined up, saying their names as they pointed to themselves, and held up one finger for one, two fingers for two. Finally they went on counting the ten Americans who should have been on the end of the line. A light began to shine in Johnny's eyes as he started to count the same way. His face lit up as he said, "Ten more! Ten more!" He turned to Thrasher and asked, "Ten more? Not all here. Where they are now?"

The group shouted, "We don't know, Johnny. We've been asking you about them."

He looked at them incredulously and said, "Others?" He slowly swept his hand along the length of their line. "I don't know where are more Americans."

Thrasher's face turned as red as a stoplight. He became visibly angry, and Jens feared for a moment that he was going to choke the kid. Instead, he dropped to the ground, pounding, kicking, and yelling. Thrasher's violent reaction, the relief of knowing that Johnny finally understood, and the realization that the group had followed this willing young Albanian with neither of them knowing what the other had in mind was just too much to bear at the moment, and Jens broke into hysterical laughter. The whole response lasted about a minute; then silence returned.

Baggs sat down and quietly explained their wishes to Johnny again.

"Okay!" Johnny said, then motioned that they should move on.

At the first few houses they came to, Johnny seemed to engage in endless conversation with the inhabitants. Some of the villagers tried to talk to the Americans. They had not seen or heard of any other Americans but weren't going to miss the opportunity to look at and talk with these.

The Italians who had been following them the day before must have gone in another direction when they heard the gunfire at Matishave. It's small wonder that the Ballista, or whoever they were, fired on us, Jens thought. We must have looked like a small army approaching that hill. The Americans were very glad that the Italians had taken another route.

The sunshine and brisk air seemed even fresher to them after having been pinned down by gunfire the day before. Shortly after noon they arrived at a cluster of houses. Johnny tried to get them some food, without success, but at least they drank water and rested. Jens was beginning to feel very hungry and was sure the others felt the same. It was Wednesday and they had had no food since Sunday in Berat.

They set out again and at 1700 they arrived at Bargulla, a village of seven houses nestled on a small plateau. It was getting dark and cold and Jens hoped the villagers would take them in to a warm fire and perhaps even a cup of some kind of hot tea. The usual crowd of the curious turned out—to look them over rather than greet them. Little girls aged six or seven stood busily knitting while listening to the conversations, scarcely glancing at their work.

Johnny talked to the village elder for at least thirty minutes, then returned to the group and in a matter-of-fact manner told Thrasher, "Other Americans here two nights."

The group bombarded him with questions. "Are you sure?" "Two nights ago or for two nights?" "How many?"

Johnny talked to the village elder again, then said, "Other Americans say too, 'Where other Americans?'"

The party laughed with relief.

The elder made known that there were at least ten Americans, maybe more, and gestured in the direction of their departure. The group decided to leave immediately and hike all night if necessary, in order to catch up. But the elder not only indicated that it would take all night to reach the next village but snarled and snapped to warn them of wolves on the trail. And so, greatly relieved to know the others had not been killed or wounded in the German attack, and with renewed confidence that they would all be reunited soon, the group stayed at the village and washed down chunks of cornbread with water before falling into sound sleep.

18 November 1943, Thursday—0600: En Route to Dobrusha

As if by consensus, several in the party awakened early and roused the others. In the half-light of dawn they grabbed their packs and slid out quietly, hoping to gain a couple of hours on their comrades.

The narrow path they followed soon climbed steeply along a switch-back trail. It was an exhausting ascent, and they stopped every few minutes to catch their breath. Jens felt grateful to the elder who had talked them out of trying this route at night. The mountains all around them were high and jagged, much like those they had flown over almost a week ago. The dysentery Jens had suffered in Sicily had returned, adding to the fatigue of hiking on an empty stomach.

It took them three hours to ascend one peak, and as they started downward again, Jens hoped the other Americans had not reached level land that would put more distance between them if they were pushing ahead.

As they neared the bottom of the trail, several houses came into view. Johnny wanted to stop for food and rest. No one objected, since by then they were all famished. The villagers who poured out of their houses as the party approached provided goat milk cheese and cornbread, which everyone devoured with relish. They left immediately afterward, and by 1800 they could see houses in the distance. They had been walking for twelve hours, and Jens was sure it would be pitch-dark before they reached this village, since it was located halfway up the next mountain. They trudged on in silence. It took all their energy just to put one foot in front of the other and to watch the trail as night settled over the jagged terrain.

The villagers put them up in several houses. The Americans had gotten a bit braver now about being separated, because it meant more space and a little more food. Jens settled herself on the floor and like everyone else took off her shoes and socks, hoping to ease the pain from hours of walking. She lay down by the fire and immediately fell asleep. A little later she was roused by Fran.

"Wake up! Food is here. Aren't you hungry?"

Jens was pleasantly surprised to find a hot meal—a kind of stew with very little meat but plenty of big, white beans. Do you suppose beans always tasted this good? Jens asked herself. She was too tired for conversation; when she finished eating, she lay back down and immediately dropped off to sleep again.

19 November 1943, Friday—0615: En Route to Dobrusha

The group was on the trail before 0630, hoping that the early start would help them catch up to their companions. After two hours, they reached another small village of six houses. An elderly man came out to greet them, and he and Johnny talked so long that members of the party looked for rocks and tree stumps to sit on while they waited. Finally Johnny returned and spoke directly to Thrasher.

"Americans stay here," Johnny said.

After much questioning, it was determined that their comrades had been at the village two nights earlier.

"Steffa here too, with American friends," Johnny said.

The group clapped, and several jumped up and down with excitement. The old man grabbed Johnny's arm and spoke to him in whispered tones. His expression told Jens that whatever he was telling Johnny was a serious matter. Finally the old man looked directly at the group and tried to communicate.

"Steffa," the old man said. He shook his head and finger, struggling to make a point.

The Americans looked at Johnny for help. "What is he trying to tell us?"

"He wants you to know that Steffa is a bad man," Johnny said. "He says Steffa friend of Germani and will turn you over to them."

"I just can't believe that," Jens said. "I stayed at his home and met his family. They seemed to have Albania's interests at heart."

"Isn't that the way most traitors would act to your face?" Elna said.

"Why didn't he stay in Berat, then?" Tassy asked. "He could have turned all of us over to the Germans. Maybe this man has a personal grudge against him." She shrugged. "Anyway, we'd better find our friends fast. If Steffa really is a supporter of the Germans, he may be leading them around, looking for Germans to turn them over to." Tassy looked and sounded worried.

"Do you suppose he urged them to go on with him instead of hiding with us?" Elna asked.

Everyone wanted to set out immediately, but the old man detained Johnny with more conversation. He offered to feed them, but they declined.

"Thank him for us," Baggs said. "But we want to cover as much territory as possible before it gets dark."

Johnny finally motioned for the party to follow him and took off as if he knew where they were going.

After another two hours at a breathless pace on the trail, Johnny pointed toward a long, low building snuggled against a hillside. There were two smaller buildings nearby.

Johnny managed to explain that the building was or had been a hospital, and maybe the other Americans were there. When the group got within earshot of the building, Jean and Marky burst out the door and ran toward them, followed by Tooie, Pauleen, and the missing medics.

"They're here! They're here!" Marky yelled.

The nurses linked arms and jumped up and down in excitement and relief.

"How did you know we were here?" Tooie asked.

"We didn't," Jens said. "We've been following our guide, Johnny, for days." Jens looked at her companions and asked, "Why didn't you come up the hill to hide with us when we left the truck last Monday?" Before anyone answered, Jens was asking more questions. "Are Maness, Lytle, and Porter with you? How many of you are here?"

Steffa appeared and shook hands with everyone. Jens felt he acted less sure of himself than when they were in Berat, almost as if he were questioning whether they would accept him. Doubts flooded in as she thought of what the old man had said about Steffa.

As the women talked, they walked into the building. Along the two longest walls was a row of hospital-height beds. The place had to have been either a hospital or a barracks. The nurses' few belongings were scattered about.

"How long have you been here?" Jens asked.

"Since yesterday about this time," Marky said. "Steffa wanted to rush along to some other village, but we refused to move. We felt sure that we must be chasing each other, so we decided to stay right here. Then if you didn't appear, maybe we'd have to go back."

Tooie explained, "Steffa didn't like our decision and has been a little peeved with us, but we told him to go ahead if he was afraid to be seen with us or whatever his concerns were. For one reason or another, he stayed."

Jens didn't have the heart to tell them what they had been told about Steffa in the last village. She hoped she had misinterpreted the comments and Steffa's actions.

19 November 1943, Friday—1330:
XII Air Force, APO 650, Foggia, Italy

Memorandum:
To: Commanding General, Twelfth Air Force, APO 650
From: XII Troop Carrier Command, APO 760

Attention is invited to enclosed Missing Air Crew Report.
For the Commanding General,
William H. Kennley, 1st Lt., Air Corps, Acting Asst. Adj. Gen.

19 November 1943, Friday—1500:
Dobrusha

"There's a nice running stream nearby," Jean said. "We've all had baths, washed our hair, and some of our clothes." She stepped forward and sniffed the air. "In fact, you downright stink, now that I'm so clean."

Jens laughed. "Okay, I can take a hint. Where is this lovely stream?"

Jean, Tooie, and Pauleen led the way. As they sat washing themselves and their clothes, they never stopped talking.

Jens wanted to know more about Steffa. "Where did Steffa want to take you?" she asked. "And why didn't you come up the side of the mountain with us, and get away from the truck when those planes came over? Didn't you hear Baggs call for all of us to follow him?"

"I heard," Jean said. "But Steffa shouted for everyone to get back on the truck so we could get to the next village quickly. He said he had friends there." Jean frowned. "I realized too late that not everybody had followed Steffa."

"Steffa told you to get back on the truck?" Jens asked.

"Yeah," Marky said. "And the Germans swooped down and strafed it."

"We heard that," Tassy said. "Were you on the truck at the time?"

"We had just jumped off," Marky said. "We were trying desperately to reach some nearby bushes so we could get out of sight."

"It was an awful feeling to see those planes drop lower all the time," Jean said. "I was afraid they'd follow the strafing by dropping a bomb."

"Did they hit the truck?" Jens asked.

"Oh, yes! Bullets splattered all around us in the bushes," Marky said. "I still don't know why no one was hit. The bullets were really close." She took a deep breath. "By that time we were almost at the village, but they couldn't get the truck restarted, so we ran the rest of the way."

"When we reached the village, we sat on a doorstep in the sun and congratulated ourselves for surviving a close brush with death or serious wounds," Jean said. "All of a sudden we heard a rumbling noise and saw dust flying in the distance. One of the men yelled, 'German tanks!' and we headed for the back of the house. Actually they were half-tracks. We could see them real well as they got closer. We all crossed our fingers, hoping they wouldn't stop, but we decided not to wait and see. We took off down a trail that a donkey would have had trouble on, let alone anything with wheels or treads."

Pauleen continued the story. "We stopped to regroup as soon as we were out of sight of the village. That's when we realized that there were only ten of us, but we couldn't go back. The half-tracks were in the village. We could only wonder which way the rest of you might go and whether you were all together."

"Has Steffa been asking about the other three girls?" Jens asked.

"Yes, but none of us know what has happened to them," Marky said. "Steffa said their 'family' would take care of them. But who knows, with the Germans in Berat?"

"On top of everything, I couldn't shake the feeling that Steffa was telling us only what he wanted us to know," Jean said.

Jens related what the village elder had told about Steffa. Suddenly Tooie and Jean were talking of incidents that could well substantiate the old man's accusations.

"Did Steffa ever say what happened to the help we were supposed to get in Berat?" Jens asked.

"Not to my knowledge," Jean said.

"Have you had food here?" Jens asked.

"Several men who seem to be caretakers of the place have brought us food when Steffa asked for it," Marky said. "How long they'll keep it up for such a large crowd is another matter."

"It's absolutely amazing that these people will share what little they have," Jens said. "We must look like a swarm of locusts when we descend on their villages. I'm sure that in most cases, they have fed us at the cost of an adequate food supply for the winter. Can you imagine thirty visitors showing up at the homes of people in the States, needing food that's been earmarked for their families? Add to that the chance of their being executed for providing those people with shelter for the night. It's a wonder that these Albanians, who have so little, are willing to risk so much for thirty people they don't know and don't expect to see ever again."

"It is amazing," Tooie agreed.

"I don't think we'll have to worry about food here much longer. I'm pretty sure Steffa will press for us to move on to the next village," Jean remarked. "He's been unusually restless here, and he's already bending the pilots' ears."

It became chilly as the sun disappeared, and the group moved inside to eat and discuss their plight in more detail. There seemed to be no immediate help in sight, and for the moment their primary concern was to remain out of German or Ballista hands.

Finally Steffa spoke up. "There are British in the country, helping the Albanians organize the partisans. I'm sure they can make contact with their headquarters in Italy or North Africa. All we have to do is get word to them about the crash and your need to get out of the country, and they'll notify the American authorities."

"Where are they located? Is it the general Hassan spoke of earlier?" Tooie asked.

"Maybe a general," Steffa said. "I'm not sure of their rank. Where they are is something we'll need to find out. Like us, they keep moving to stay out of German hands."

"Could we send a runner with a message to find them?" Marky asked.

"I wish we had thought of this earlier," Lois said.

"We can't undo the past," Marky said. "But maybe we can do something about our future."

"Does anyone have some paper we can write a note on?" Lois asked.

"I have," Jens said. "What should we put in the message?"

"The type, ID number of the plane, and the date we crashed should start it off," Baggs said in his Georgia drawl. "We can sign it with the pilot's initials. That way if this runner gets caught, we haven't confirmed anything for the Krauts."

Steffa obtained a runner from the village, repeated the final instructions for him, and handed him the scrap of paper that would tell the British what had happened and the group's probable moves. Spirits soared as they realized there was a real possibility of getting word to the outside and finding help to get back to their own lines.

"How long will it take a runner to make the trip?" Tassy asked.

"Who knows?" Thrasher said. "It depends how far he has to go to find the British. Then he'll have to get back to us with their reply." He shrugged. "We'll just have to wait and see."

"Can we wait here for him?" Marky asked.

Steffa spoke up immediately. "We cannot wait here. It would be too dangerous. This place is too open and too well known to the Germans and Ballista. We need to reach a higher altitude where the villages are less accessible. It's not so easy for an enemy to reach these places in force, since they have to be approached on foot or horseback."

"Do you think the Germans know we're here?" Jean asked.

Steffa smiled. "Not right here maybe, but now that they have Berat, I'm sure they know you're in the area."

"I can't believe the Germans are so interested in a bunch of medical personnel," Sergeant Adams said.

"They may have heard, as we did, that you are some kind of invasion force," Steffa said.

"What happened to the help we were supposed to get in Berat?" Jens asked. She watched Steffa closely for his response.

Steffa looked puzzled. "I know of no one in Berat who could have been of aid to you. If Hassan had known of anyone, surely he would have made contact."

It sounds fishy to me, Jens thought, but she was not willing to confront him further just yet.

6 The Enemy Closes In

20 November 1943, Saturday—0710: En route to Derzhezha.

Jens awakened early and was happy to walk to the stream to brush her teeth and wash her face. It was a luxury after weeks on the trail with no facilities for personal sanitation.

When she returned, the Americans were saying goodbye to Johnny and thanking him for his help. He was taking a different trail than they would. Jens felt sorry to see Johnny go. She believed that he had genuinely wanted to help them and had no hidden agendas.

At 1000 hours they grabbed their gear and followed Steffa at a leisurely pace. Whenever they met people along the trail, Steffa would have long conversations with them. The party could always tell when he informed the people that his charges were Americans. Usually there were audible gasps, followed by the exclamation "Americano!" Whatever else he told them was anyone's guess, but he always picked up word about the movements of the Germans and Ballista. How much of that information was fact and how much rumor, neither Steffa nor the Americans had any way of knowing for sure. There was considerably more serenity in being with someone who could ask the questions they constantly had and who could tell them what information he had received. Once again Jens was certain that Steffa was a staunch partisan, yet she couldn't mesh that fact with his leaving his wife and five children at the mercy of the Germans. Was it because his family was at no risk from an army that he cooperated with whenever possible? Perhaps he thought the Germans would not harm his family as long as he wasn't present. Then again, maybe he was just looking after his own hide.

During a rest period, while the group sat on rocks enjoying the sunshine, Steffa suggested that since they had no particular destination for the day, they might head for one of the villages at a higher elevation which the people along the road had told him about. Perhaps they could rest there for a day or two, depending on the shelter and food available. Everyone in the party quickly agreed and started off again after fifteen minutes of rest.

The trail they were following was no more than a narrow shelf, chopped out of the mountainside, which switched back and forth as it ascended at a very steep angle. The air was clear, brisk, and slightly thinner as they gained altitude. It took two exhausting hours of climbing to reach the top. Jens had expected a spectacular view; instead, she saw other high mountains pressing against the peak they had just climbed, and the tortuous trail that led down the other side of the crest.

The descent was just as challenging as the climb. Jens longed for a handrail or at least a few bushes along the edge to help her negotiate the steep incline. At the bottom ran ribbonlike along the floor of the valley a stream that hugged its way through a gorge and fell from a mountain cliff far above them. The group decided the stream was well filtered and free from typhoid, so they bent to drink their fill of the cold, clean water, then filled their canteens. The trail was narrow, however, and they were forced to climb again.

By 1400 the sun was hidden behind the massive mountains. The sky overhead was clear and dark. The party followed Steffa and the newly acquired village guides single file up the steep flank of the mountain, reminding Jens of a flock of baby ducks following their mother. They walked without conversation because the demands of the climb took all the breath they had and turned the already painful act of walking into a real battle. They stopped every fifteen minutes to force air into their oxygen-starved lungs, and in the silent majesty of the mountains the only noise they heard was the sound of their own labored breathing.

"Steffa was sure right about this place," Sergeant Allen said between gasps. "I'd be willing to bet that God alone knows for sure that it exists, and it's for damn sure the Germans won't be traveling up here in any kind of force. In fact, I doubt any of them would want to make this climb."

It was almost dark when they arrived at the village of Derzhezha. Dogs barked, and people spilled out of the town's seven houses. Given the climb they had gone through to reach their destination, Jens concluded that the village probably received very few visitors. Two elderly men approached the party and after greeting them, began speaking to Steffa. The conversation went on so long, Jens began to doubt they'd be granted shelter. She felt sure she could sleep on the stone wall where she was sitting and assured herself that would be preferable to negotiating the trail in the dark. Finally, Steffa told the Americans that the villagers had very little food but were willing to shelter the party for the night and provide what food they could. The group's hopes for spending several days resting in Derzhezha vanished, however. It was damp and getting very cold. The nurses removed the liners from their trench coats and gave them to the sergeants for the night as they broke into small groups and left for the individual houses that would be their homes for the evening.

21 November 1943, Sunday—0700:
En Route to Leshnija

Early the next morning an Albanian who Jens figured must be the village elder came and sat down on the floor next to Steffa. He talked about fifteen minutes before Steffa turned to the nurses.

"The people are sorry they cannot offer you a place to rest for several days," Steffa said. "But they have barely enough food for themselves for the winter."

"Please tell them we understand, and thank them for their kindnesses last night," Jens said.

Steffa turned again to the elder, and the two talked for another ten minutes before he spoke in English again.

"We shall be leaving shortly," Steffa said. "When you have your

things together, go to the square. We'll gather and leave from there."
He stood up. "I'll go now and tell the rest of our group."

"Where are we going? And how far is it?" Fran Nelson asked
before Steffa could get out the door. She had been so quiet since the
two groups were reunited that her questions startled Jens.

"This man has been asking guides from the town to lead us to
the next village," Steffa said. "It's about a five-hour walk from here,
maybe a little more for you, since you're not in good walking condition."

"You can say that again," Jens said. "But why that particular
village? Is there someone there who can help us?"

"No," Steffa said. "I know of no one to help us now. But this
gentleman says the Ballista are very active in areas we just came
through, so we can't go back. All we can do is move about, seeking
shelter and food until we hear from the British. It is very isolated in
these mountains, so at least we are safe here."

As they walked along the trail, climbing their way carefully,
Jens hoped they would find a stream so she could brush her teeth.

The temperature fell as the party climbed higher, and a cold,
bone-chilling wind whipped at their inadequate clothing and fought
their inch-by-inch progress. The drop in temperature had one ben-
eficial effect: it numbed their aching feet and dulled the pain that
had become an integral part of every step they took. It was almost
dark when the Americans labored up the steep trail to the secluded
village of Leshnija.

Most of them were suffering from dysentery by now, with violent cramps and diarrhea. There had been many occasions in the
almost six-hour hike when individuals had to run behind bushes in
order to accommodate their symptoms. Everyone was chagrined that
there was no paper to help with sanitation.

Jens had become proficient in assessing the accommodations a
village could offer, just by seeing the houses that made it up. As she
looked over this tiny hamlet of six rough stone houses, she concluded
that it would be a cold night—the windows of the houses had neither
glass nor shutters—and that most likely there would be no food, though
with luck there might be cornbread. Jens didn't feel very hungry and
thought perhaps her body was adjusting to the near-starvation diet.

She sat down on a rock and put her head on her knees, waiting for housing arrangements to be made; it seemed to be taking forever. Even a dirt floor would look good right now, she thought. Surely they'll take us in for the night, even if they can't feed us. If not, I'll just sleep right here. I don't think any of us could make it to the next village at night, especially not me.

She watched Steffa as he talked to a group of village men. Every fifteen minutes or so he'd return to Thrasher and Baggs and report his progress. Jens moved to a rock closer to the pilots so she could hear the conversation. In minutes, she learned that the enemy, whether Germans or Ballista or a combination of both, had been raiding villages fairly close by. The village had had a scouting party out all day to determine where their enemies were and where they were heading, but as the scouts hadn't returned yet, the situation remained very unclear. Steffa seemed to think the danger was mainly from the Ballista, but Ballista or Germans, the enemy was afoot, and the villagers didn't seem keen on taking the chance that an enemy raiding party might find them sheltering Americans. After another long conversation, with Steffa doing most of the talking, the villagers agreed to keep them for the night, and they were quickly assigned to various houses until morning.

"Another cold one tonight," Sergeant Zeiber said as he accepted the liner from Jens's trench coat.

"I'm afraid so. Just don't forget to pick up my liner as you leave if we get routed in a hurry during the night," Jens told him.

"Did it sound that bad?" Zeiber asked.

"I guess no one knows for sure until that scouting party returns, if they do get back with their skins and scalps," Jens said. She shivered and her teeth chattered audibly. She wondered if she were just cold or getting the chills.

The house was dingier than any they'd been in before and a stark contrast to Steffa's home in Berat. The five nurses assigned to it sat down by the fire and pulled off soggy shoes and socks. Jens looked at the soles of her GI oxfords and felt sure they couldn't stay intact much longer, especially since they got soaked daily. She placed her shoes near the fire to dry and laid her socks over them. The socks were stiff with dirt but still holding up without holes. No one seemed to be in the mood for conversation, and Jens lay down on the floor, crooked her arms under her head, and closed her eyes. She was aware that the floor was thick with dirt, dust, and debris, but such things mattered little now, and in less than five minutes she was fast asleep.

When she awakened hours later, cold and stiff, she guessed that no one had been in to see them or to offer them food, since none of her companions for the night had awakened her. Everyone was sleeping soundly, and the fire was almost out. She crawled around the room looking for more wood, but to no avail. Shivering and shaking with cold, she realized that she needed to go to the toilet, but had fallen asleep without learning its location. In most of the places where they had stayed, the host merely opened the back door and waved his hand to indicate that the toilet was anywhere outside that a person chose. That might well be the case here, but there were added complications. With the enemy in the area, the villagers might well have posted guards around the houses, and those guards might be trigger-happy. She lay down, curled up, and tried to visualize herself as warm and comfortable. According to her watch it was 0500. Daylight can't be too far away, she thought, not even this late in November.

Just as the first sign of light appeared in the sky an Albanian walked into the room, carrying several pieces of wood. He looked at the barely living fire, shook his head, and chided the Americans in Albanian. His facial expression and tone of voice said it all. Somehow he was angry at his visitors for not maintaining the fire—despite the fact that there was no wood available to them. Later Jens learned that there were no matches in the village. If a fire went out, it required a flame from an ongoing fire to restart the one that had died. She concluded that the man's anger was, in fact, frustration and displaced blame.

Their host sat on the floor, fed the smoldering ashes with small pieces of bark, and blew on the small glow until it became a flame, then expanded into a blaze.

Jens asked the man the location of the toilet and followed him to a door that opened onto the wide expanse lying behind the tiny stone house. He waved his hand in a sweeping motion, and she nodded and smiled to indicate that she understood. Her host returned to the fire and Jens decided to get company for her trip to the "ladies' room." Jean was sitting up.

"Have you seen the bathroom yet?" Jens asked.

"Yes," Jean answered. "Large, isn't it?"

"How would one of you like to accompany me to a small spot before it gets lighter and there are more people around?" she asked.

"We might as well all go," Jean said.

The five women stepped out the door into thick, black mud. Jens led, picking her way around what looked like dry clumps of dirt or stone. Suddenly one clump leaped up and ran away before she could get her foot solidly planted. It was a big black sheep. She had barely regained her balance when other almost indiscernible creatures stirred, stood up, and meandered away from the intruders. White sheep were becoming visible as Jens's eyes adjusted to the half-light of morning fog, but the black ones blended right into the dark earth.

Twenty minutes later their host passed a tray of cornbread and allowed fifteen minutes for breakfast. Then he opened the front door and, with a sweep of his right arm, bowed the Americans out of his house.

The group reassembled and as usual, compared notes on bed and board before the conversation changed to a newer topic—the whereabouts of the enemy. They looked for Steffa and saw that he was engrossed in conversation with three village men.

Fran Nelson stood bent over, her head barely visible inside the hood of her trench coat. "I wish the sun had the decency to shine on my poor aching back. I might get it straightened out again." She chuckled. "I was curled up into a ball all night trying to keep warm; now I'm afraid my back may stay curved like a pretzel."

"With or without the sun, you'll be plenty warm when we start hiking again," Lois Watson said.

"What's the holdup anyway?" Sergeant Allen bellowed.

Steffa came over and spoke in his usual quiet voice.

"We're waiting for special guides."

"I thought that was arranged last night," Tooie said.

"It was," Steffa answered. "But we learned late that the Ballista have moved into a village on our route, so we'll have to go over that mountain." He pointed toward a high, jagged peak. "The villagers here say they don't know the mountain trails well enough to take us, so last night they sent for some guides from another village. They should be here any minute."

The group looked at the mountain and began to size it up. They had already crossed so many mountains, they felt like experts.

"It doesn't look too bad from here," Sergeant Hayes said. "That is, if we're seeing all of it."

Suddenly Steffa started down the trail, and the party saw a young boy and two men approaching the village. Jens wondered if they had brought word concerning enemy movements in the area. After what seemed to her to be a violent argument, the conversation stopped, and the men said goodbye in the usual Muslim fashion of touching their hands to their hearts and bowing slightly.

Jens hurried over to Steffa. "What's the word?" she asked. "Can we go on? Did the guides get here yet? Are the Germans and Ballista close by?"

"They say it's safe," Steffa said.

Jens felt a flash of anger. She wanted to jump on Steffa and beat him about the head, yelling, "Tell us every word that was said! There has to be more information!" Steffa's unspoken refusal to tell them everything was increasing their distrust. They began trying to interpret his every movement, word, and facial expression. Those few derogatory comments spoken to them by the elderly villager had planted the seeds of suspicion that Steffa might possibly betray them to the enemy.

7 Blizzard on the Mountain

22 November 1943, Monday—1015: Mount Tomorrit

It was midmorning as the Americans began their hike to Terlioria. Between them and the village lay Mount Tomorrit. At 8,136 feet in altitude, it was one of the highest peaks in Albania, and with the cold drizzle that had just begun the climb promised to be anything but easy or comfortable. The beginning of the trail ascended gently up the side of the barren mountain. In the light rain and persistent overcast the landscape looked brown and gray, and the wet earth soaked quickly through Jens's worn shoes. She hoped that the growing numbness from the cold would soon ease her foot pain, as it had previously.

As they climbed, the temperature dropped; the rain turned to sleet, then snow, adding to an already miserable situation. The precipitation made the ground slippery and progress slow. Jens peered out from her hood at the terrain ahead. She saw an open, barren plateau that stretched out to snow-covered mountains. The trail turned sharply to the right as fine snow swirled about their heads and a bitter cold wind sucked the breath from their lungs. Without warning, a large black cloud slipped over a ridge and hung menacingly above them. Soon the group was enveloped in violent cold wind and blinding snow. Jens realized that she could no longer see the person in front of her, and their tracks in the snow were covered so quickly that they were impossible to follow. The snow spun in circles and beat at her face with such force that taking a deep breath was not possible. She tried to call to one of the men directly ahead of her, but the wind drove her words back into her mouth. She knew that half of the party was behind her and turned to see if they were still following. Marky and Fran almost walked over her.

Jens's fingers felt frozen inside her wet leather gloves. She believed if she could remove her gloves, she could rub her hands together to warm them, but her numb fingers would not obey her command. She pushed her hands deep into her trench coat pockets but found that she needed her arms free to maintain her balance. She began to walk faster, attempting to keep the person ahead of her in sight, hoping that person could see someone who was following the guides, praying that the guides knew the trail well, since all landmarks must be covered with snow by this time. Jens stopped and looked behind her again, assessing the group's ability to keep up. A long-legged sergeant overtook her, and she grabbed his arm. It was Cruise, and she put her mouth next to his ear and yelled, wondering if he could hear her above the wind.

"If you catch up with the guides, slow them down! We're losing sight of one another. We could end up scattered all over this mountain."

"Yeah, that's where I'm heading, God willing," Cruise yelled into Jens's ear. His Boston accent was unmistakable even in a blizzard.

Jens thrust her hands in front of her. "Pull my gloves off," she hollered. Cruise tugged and jerked her gloves off wrong side out.

The sergeant bent forward. "Pull my hat down so it covers my ears."

Jens tugged at his hat with her numb fingers and eventually got it to cover most of Cruise's ears.

"Thanks!" he shouted above the storm. He took off in his long stride and disappeared into the curtain of snow that enveloped them.

Jens looked back just in time to see the feet of one of the nurses go out from under her. Two of the men tried to pull her up, but she seemed limp. It was Tooie.

"Get up! Get up! Don't just lie there," Jens shouted. She could barely hear her own voice.

Tooie staggered to her feet and immediately fell into a heap again. Two sergeants grabbed her under the arms and half-walked, half-dragged her up and forward. Jens turned and hurried ahead, hoping to catch sight of someone up the trail from them.

"Don't they ever look back to see if we're following? I'll skin them alive if I ever catch up with them," she muttered to herself.

Jens and her companions were encrusted with snow. She tried to move her toes, but couldn't feel them at all. Her face felt stiff as she continued to wiggle her nose and cheeks. She remembered walking to and from school during blizzards back in Duluth, Minnesota, before her family moved to Michigan. Her mother had told her and her older sister always to keep moving: "Don't think you can sit, or lie down to rest. Wiggle your nose, cheeks, fingers and toes all the time." Slipping, sliding, and fighting the gale-force winds had left her almost totally exhausted. Suddenly she ran into someone's back. She looked up and recognized Thrasher and the guides. They were standing huddled together with their backs to the wind. Cruise had caught up and persuaded them to wait for the rest of the party. Jens pushed herself tight against them and tucked her hands under her coat, close to her body. They were so numb that she couldn't tell if they moved on command or not.

The guides seemed terribly agitated and began stomping back and forth and waving their arms at the column behind them, urging them to hurry. When they were all in a tight formation again, they pushed on, and the going seemed a little easier after the brief, un-scheduled stop. The reprieve didn't last long, however, and after twenty minutes it was hard to remember there had been even that much rest.

Without warning, the guides stopped in their tracks. Jens couldn't hear a word but could see them well enough to know they were hotly debating an important matter. Are they arguing about which route to take? Jens asked herself. Suddenly a terrible thought filled her mind. Dear God, she thought, they're lost!

The snow had caused a virtual whiteout on the mountain, and there were no trail markers left uncovered. We could wander up here until we freeze to death, Jens told herself. Dear God help them find the right way. Just as suddenly as they had stopped, the guides ceased gesturing and continued straight ahead.

Jens had never felt so cold in her life. She couldn't feel her feet at all and marveled that she was still walking. She had continued to wiggle her nose and cheeks, but with every movement, she felt as if her face were cracking. In her mind she could see the fissures.

Just as suddenly as they had walked into the storm, they walked out of it. The wind was no longer howling like an animal mad with pain and rage, and the solid white curtain of swirling powder changed to gently falling flakes. The stillness and brightness were eerie. Jens looked back and saw the clearly defined edge of the black cloud, just as she had seen it before the storm began. She checked her watch and estimated that they had been in the storm about forty-five minutes. She felt certain that if it had lasted another forty-five minutes, few if any of their party would have made it off the mountain.

22 November 1943, Monday—1445: Terlioria

The trail dropped abruptly downhill, and very soon they were in slushy snow again. They followed the trail through another sharp turn and saw a small village just below them. Benumbed and exhausted, they stumbled into the town as barking dogs announced their arrival. A small cluster of men and women, capes draped around their shoulders, watched them approach, their chatter growing more excited as the weary hikers got closer. The Albanians came forward for a better view. Steffa quickly told the Americans why the villagers were excited.

"They are calling you Albanian heroes because we crossed our third highest mountain after September. No Albanians who know the danger would attempt such a climb!"

"Yeah, I believe I understand why," Baggs said.

Steffa went on to tell the villagers about their ordeal, and they quickly and graciously invited the Americans into their homes. A young girl pulled Jens's wet shoes and socks off her half-frozen feet, then brought a wooden tub of warm water and placed her feet gently into it to soak.

"Oh, thank you! Thank you," Jens said. Tears of relief and gratitude rolled down her cheeks. "You're so kind."

Later, Jean, Elna, and Jens curled up into a ball with their backs to the fire, doubting that they would ever again get warm clear through. The young girl brought them food, a very tallowy mutton stew that stuck to the roofs of their mouths but was fairly warm and had identifiable pieces of meat in it.

"That was quite a storm even by South Dakota standards," Elna said. "I had visions of someone finding our bones in the spring."

"We're lucky the blizzard was so localized," Jean said. "If it hadn't been, I doubt we'd be here talking about it now. It was amazing how quickly it moved in on us. I wondered why the guides didn't turn back."

"I guess they had no choice with the Ballista behind us," Elna said, "and those other villagers surely didn't want us back, given the circumstances. Now I know what it means to be between the devil and the deep blue sea."

A loud knock interrupted them, the outside door swung open, and the pilots and Steffa bounded into the room.

"We have words of cheer!" Baggs said. "News! Good news!" Big smiles lighted their faces, and Baggs waved a piece of paper in the air.

"News? What news? From where?" Jens asked.

"Remember our runner?" Baggs asked. "He just returned from the British."

"He did!" Elna exclaimed. "Where are the British? What did they say?"

Thrasher took the paper and began to read the message. "'Since you are heading this way, you may as well come to Lovdar, where I shall plan to meet you on 01 December, or as soon as I receive word that you are there. We can make plans for your evacuation then. Signed, Smith, British Forces.'"

"Evacuation! Doesn't that sound heavenly!" Elna exclaimed. "How far is Lovdar?"

"I don't know," Thrasher said, "but he's given us several days to get there."

"A nice benign name, 'Smith!'" Jens said. "I wonder what his real name is."

"Who cares!" Jean yelled. She threw her socks into the air. "At least we're moving in the right direction, and for a good reason."

"Wouldn't it have been hell," Baggs said, "to have the runner come to this village only to find out that we'd all perished in that damned blizzard!"

"Oh, please!" Jens exclaimed. "*Perish* the thought."

"I wonder which direction he came here from," Thrasher said. "Not the same way we came, I hope." He leaned forward. "My God! I never knew that snow could blow so hard in your face as to almost choke you! This Floridian has seen most of his snow in neatly framed pictures."

"It wasn't just the snow," Jens said. "That wind seemed to suck the breath right out of you." She looked at Baggs. "Not to mention that I was sure the guides were lost when they stopped to argue. I still think we might have gotten lucky when they decided which way to go."

"Well, maybe we'll get a few more lucky turns and finally get back to our lines," Baggs said.

"There's no 'maybe' about it," Elna said. "We will get back to our own lines. After going through a plane crash, being bombed and strafed by Germans, being shot at by Ballists, and surviving a mountain blizzard, I just can't believe that anything could keep us from getting back safely."

The group's spirits soared as they looked forward to meeting the British officer, Smith, and planning their evacuation.

8 The British Captain Smith

Memorandum:

For: Major General Smith, AFHQ

1. The following radio was received from the Air Service Command Advance Headquarters at Bari:

"Suggest that General Eisenhower CMA, the surgeon NATOUSA, CMA and Troop Carrier Command be given the following information which may or may not be known in their headquarters PD From Oboe Sugar Sugar it is learned that Middle East reported that a party of three zero Americans including one three Uncle Sugar Army Nurses are believed to be in Albania PD It is presumed here that they are attempting to reach the coast PD British plans for rescue party awaiting details on location CMA requested from Cairo Rpt Cairo PD Uncle Sugar Naval Lieutenant attached to Oboe Sugar Sugar is believed to have gone across today to the Glen party to seek information and organize search if possible PD At this Headquarters nurses referred to are believed to be from eight zero seven Air Evacuation Unit."

2. The above is a radiogram referred to in a phone conversation with Lt. Robertson.

David Stinson,

Colonel, GSC,
Chief of Staff
CC: Surgeon, NATOUSA

29 November 1943, Monday—1000:
NATOUSA, APO 534, U.S. ARMY

MEMORANDUM:
TO: CG, ARMY AIR FORCES, WASHINGTON, D.C.,
(Atten: Statistical Control Division)
Enclosure—Missing Air Crew Report.
A/C 42-68809, dated 13 November 1943, Pilot, Thrasher,
Charles B., 1st Lt. and three crew members, 26 passengers;
all non-battle casualty status.

29 November 1943, Monday—1310:
Lovdar

As the snow turned to slush and mud, the group's week-long hike over the mountains became more precarious, but now the terrain had leveled out to a large plateau with a few trees scattered here and there. Just as Sergeant Allen took a position behind Jens, he started yelling.

"Do you see those buildings up ahead? Do you see them?"

Jens turned and saw him pointing to a spot in the distance. "I see," she said. "What about them?"

"That's Lovdar!" he shouted.

"Lovdar?" Jens felt incredulous. "This isn't the first of December, how can we be at Lovdar?"

"For once, we're ahead of schedule," Allen said. He rushed off down the single file line to spread the good news.

Jens looked at the distant village and hoped the British officer named Smith would be waiting for them with information regarding their evacuation plans.

Despite the constant pain in their feet, the pace increased considerably after everyone heard the news. To her chagrin, Jens soon found herself near the end of the single file. "Darn that shoe!" she said aloud, more aware than ever that she had to pick up her foot high enough to flop the loose sole back into place.

"Just think, by tonight or tomorrow morning we'll be making concrete plans for our evacuation to our own lines," Elna said.

"Maybe the British know of a place they can bring a plane in for a landing," Jens said. "It would be nice to get air-evac'd instead of having to walk back to the coast."

"That would be great," Tooie said, "but I haven't seen any-where a plane could land in these mountains. Most likely, evacuation by sea would be easier for whoever is going to get us out."

"Putting a boat in along the Albanian coast would be no small feat," Sergeant Shumway said. He was limping and walking with a stick to ease the pain in the knee he had injured in the crash landing. "I'm sure the Germans patrol every inch of navigable coastline, and coastline where a boat could be brought in is at a real premium in Albania."

Conversation stopped as they reached the outskirts of Lovdar. Jens estimated there were probably eight to ten houses in the vil-lage. She was examining them for chimneys and their windows for glass when the party passed the second house and entered an open area where several men were standing around what she at first thought was a fountain but turned out to be a water pump. The man leaning against it straightened up slowly and watched as they approached. In a second or two Jens recognized the British uniform. The officer was a young blond man of average height. It's Smith, Jens thought. He's here already! The officer seemed to be considering whether the motley group limping toward him could be the Americans he had come to rescue. Suddenly he stepped toward them at a brisk pace, with a hand outstretched. He smiled broadly as each American tried to shake his hand and spoke a word or two of greeting. They could scarcely believe he was real, barely believe they were finally going to get help from the Allies.

"I'm Captain Smith," the officer said in a quiet voice, and un-mistakable British accent.

"Captain Smith," Jens said, "you have no idea how good you look to us."

"Has it been a terribly hard journey so far?" Smith asked.

"Well—" Jens said, "it hasn't exactly been a stroll through the park. The past ten days have been the most rugged, but as long as our feet hold out, I guess we'll make it."

For a moment or two, the group just stared at him as if afraid he might disappear if he weren't within their sight. Then the pilots stepped forward and talked with him for several minutes before he motioned for the whole group to gather closer. They squeezed around him and stood waiting without a whisper.

The captain began to speak. "We're going to put you up here for now. My colleagues and I are in the next village which is nearby. We feel it's prudent not to stay together, so if for any reason we have to leave in a hurry, we'll have a better chance of getting away safely." He smiled. "But don't worry about it. We've been left here peacefully for some time, but of course, we need to take precautions." He paused and looked around the group. "The first thing I shall need is a list of your full names, rank, and serial numbers. We shall try to let your air corps know that we have all of you."

"All of us?" Jens asked. "Have you heard from the other three?"

Smith looked surprised. "Other three—are there more of you?"

"Yes, three of our nurses were separated from us when we fled Berat," Baggs said.

"Fled Berat?" Smith asked. "How long ago was that?"

"November fifteenth," Baggs answered. "We thought maybe when you heard about us, you might have heard about them too."

"We didn't know of your existence until we received the note you sent by runner a week ago." Smith looked very sincere. He spoke kindly. "I'm sorry. We've had no word of them to this point. Please add their names and other information to the written list I've requested." His tone became lighter. "The village people have agreed to take you in and, in fact, seem eager to meet young Americans."

"Eager to meet us?" Jens asked. "Things are getting too good to be true."

"How long will we be here?" Sergeant Allen asked.

Smith smiled patiently. "Maybe two or three days. We shall have to wait and see how things develop."

Jens looked from Captain Smith's clean, neat uniform to her

own. Her clothes and those of her companions were filthy and be-
draggled.

Smith talked again to the pilots for several minutes, then turned
his attention back to the group. "There are people here now to take
you to their homes."

The nurses were placed five to a house. As they entered the low
building, Jens was struck by its being truly a home. They were in a
comfortable room with a big stone fireplace and two large glass windows that let the light in and made the room bright. On either side
of the fireplace were low, wide beds with pillows propped up against
the wall. Each bed could easily sleep three. A woman and young girl
asked them in sign language and a few words the nurses recognized
if they would like a bath.

"A bath? Po, po!" Tooie exclaimed in her recently acquired Albanian for "yes."

They nodded vigorously and motioned to ask if they could wash
their hair too. The woman didn't seem to approve of that, probably
because they'd have to sleep with wet hair, the nurses decided, and it
was too cold for that.

The lady of the house seemed delighted that her guests were so
pleased with her efforts. She left the room and was gone at least
thirty minutes. Suddenly a door in the back of the room burst open,
and their hostess ushered in a man carrying a round, shallow wooden
tub, which he placed in front of the fire. The squeals of delight
brought a bright smile to the woman's face, though the nurses were
amused that the woman could think any of them would fit into the
small tub. The man left, and the young girl appeared with large pitchers of hot and cold water.

"Who goes first? And who has some soap left?" Tooie asked.

"I won't mind being a guinea pig for this process," Jens responded. She was the tallest of the five and if she could bathe in the
tub, any of them would fit.

The woman motioned for them to disrobe. As they undressed,
the woman and girl looked amazed to see only a brassiere under
their shirts. They clasped their hands about their bodies and shivered for the Americans. As Jens dropped her clothes on the bed, the
older woman grabbed them up and walked to the other side of the

room. She examined the shirt and battle jacket, turning the seams out and looking at them closely. Jens realized that the woman was looking for body lice, and she felt sure she would discover them, as they had often found the pests themselves. Jens thoroughly understood that their hostess would not want body lice in her beds.

The tub was so small that each bather had to sit with her knees drawn up under her chin; nevertheless, they found the warm water a true luxury. Without a word, the young girl lifted each nurse's legs out of the water and scrubbed them with the washcloth Jens had produced from her musette bag. Jens was convinced that if the girl had had a scrub brush, she would have used it to get the dirt and grime off of them.

The American guests were pleasantly surprised at being served a supper of mutton, rice, and cornbread, a truly tasty meal. Five minutes after eating they were in bed and sinking comfortably into the soft feather mattress. Jens was certain that she would sleep immediately and was taken off guard when, instead, her thoughts turned to Lytle, Maness, and Porter. With some of the ordinary necessities of life taken care of, help at hand, and evacuation imminent, she wondered where they were and why no one knew what had happened to them. She feared more than ever that they had been captured in Berat. Tears rolled down her cheeks as she considered her present comfort and thought of what they might be going through at that very minute.

30 November 1943, Tuesday—0815: Lovdar

The five nurses awakened after daylight and enjoyed the luxury of lying in bed and talking. The day was overcast, but there was no rain or snow. The young girl, Nadia, brought in cornbread and tea on a tray. After breakfast, the wooden tub and pitchers of hot and cold water reappeared. They shampooed their hair with the little soap they had left, and Nadia poured warm water over their heads to rinse the soap away. The small, thin towel that Jens took from her musette bag didn't dry much, and she was glad that her thick brown hair was very short. She sat in front of the fire and tousled it until it was dry.

By noon the women were more relaxed than they had been since their plane ran into that storm on its way to Bari. The nurses asked about washing their clothes, but Nadia, who looked to be about fifteen, insisted on washing them herself. Her guests would have liked to talk with her, but since they knew so little Albanian, all they could do was smile and thank her profusely.

30 November 1943, Tuesday—1300: OSS Advance Base, Bari, Italy

Captain Lloyd G. Smith, a twenty-four-year-old intelligence officer with the Office of Strategic Services (OSS) received orders from the Commanding Officer, Advance Base, Bari, to proceed to Albania to bring out an American party that had crash-landed near Elbasan on 8 November 1943. Smith was told that the party was thought to be heading for the southwest coast. His mission was to learn the whereabouts of the Americans, make contact with them, and bring them to the coast for evacuation by sea.

30 November 1943, Tuesday—1400: Lovdar

Jens's dysentery returned worse than ever, with nausea and severe abdominal cramping. She longed for a real inside bathroom but had to make do with an outhouse that resembled an American "two-holer." At least, she thought, it's better than having to use the great outdoors. But she made so many trips across the soggy ground that her shoes stayed wet. Between trips, she lay on the bed lulled by the crackling of the fire. If she hadn't been suffering those disruptive and uncomfortable symptoms, she easily could have spent the day sleeping.

Early that evening the pilots visited for about an hour. They were clean, relaxed, and partially shaved. They had each decided to grow a mustache and Thrasher had tried to fashion his dark beard into a goatee. They had come with the news that the mayor of the village was planning to give a supper in honor of these American visitors.

Just hearing the word "supper" made Jens more nauseated. The pain in her abdomen was right under her ribs and severe enough to make her wish that she had codeine, but they had run out of it the previous week. They had plenty of morphine of course, but she felt its use would be extreme.

Her four roommates, having finally gotten their hair combed and their make-up on, left for the mayor's house. Jens was too sick to go even for tea. As she lay in the room alone, her thoughts turned to the rest of the 807th in Sicily. By now they must know that Jens and her companions were still alive. She could imagine their surprise when they learned that the rest of the squadron was stranded in German-occupied Albania. Her thoughts turned to battle casualties, and she wondered if the patient load had increased with all the Allied activity in Italy. If so, the members of the 807th remaining in Sicily would be doing double and triple duty. Jens felt sure that the commanding officer at Catania would never allow so many members of the squadron to fly on the same plane again.

Despite her pain and nausea, she felt glad that since the Allies now knew where they were and that they were in relatively good health, her parents wouldn't be told she was missing. In fact, she thought, the letter I wrote before we left is probably just arriving. At least my parents won't have to go through weeks of worry about what has happened to us.

01 December 1943, Wednesday—0930: En Route to Krushove

The British Captain Smith returned to Lovdar in the morning. He announced that he had decided to take the group to the village where he and his associates were staying so they could care for them better and make faster progress with evacuation plans.

"It isn't very far," Smith said, "but it is at a higher altitude, so if you can gather your things quickly and come with me, we can easily be there before dark."

Jens was very glad that her pain, nausea, and dysentery were gone for the moment. She and the others stuffed their belongings into their musette bags, grabbed their coats, thanked their hostess again, and followed Smith out of the house.

The party had been walking for over an hour when Sergeant Allen asked Captain Smith how long it would take to reach their destination.

Captain Smith laughed. "I can't say exactly how long it will take you, but I can say that I came over here in about three and a half hours today."

The snow was getting deeper with every step—so deep that even the men over six feet tall were frequently in snow up to their waists. Occasionally, members of the party stepped into a hole and found themselves in snow to their underarms. Jens felt weak with exhaustion after her miserable day and night of cramps, nausea, and diarrhea. It occurred to her that if she dropped farther back in line, more of the group would have tramped through, making the trail easier. Stepping slightly off the trail, she allowed several tall sergeants to go on ahead of her and then found the walking slightly easier. She thanked God that the trail was not a narrow one and made note of the fact that they were gradually climbing higher; the temperature was growing colder and the air thinner.

She turned to look behind her as she heard men's voices calling, "Get up! Get up!" and recognized Sergeant Allen lying spread-eagled in the snow. Two of the other men had taken hold of his arms and were pulling him to his feet. She waited for them to catch up.

"We're almost there, Allen. Don't give up now," Bob Owen coaxed.

Allen flopped to his side and moaned. "This snow is paralyzing my legs. They're so cold, they're cramping." It was unlike Allen to give up, but now he was whimpering and holding his legs. "They ache. They're cramping. I can't stand up."

Two of the tallest sergeants tried to carry him between them on their hands, but the deep snow made their efforts futile.

Finally the six-foot-two Owen bent down and said, "Crawl on my back," and carried him piggyback for a while, rubbing Allen's legs as he walked.

Technical Sergeant Paul G. Allen was the liveliest in the group and had saved the day many times with his entertaining storytelling. Jens was certain that the tales were all manufactured, despite the fact that Allen told them in the first person. She had howled at these yarns, and Allen soon learned which individuals were his best audience; he always managed to get within earshot of those people. He seemed to know instinctively whenever a story—true, false, or exaggerated—was needed most. His snub nose and the shock of hair that stuck out from under his knit cap made him look even younger than his age, so in spite of his derring-do attitude he aroused the protective instincts of everyone in the party.

The rubbing, and perhaps the warmth of Owen's body, must have warmed Allen pretty well, for after thirty-five minutes he got down, determined to walk the rest of the way on his own two feet.

Jens looked at her watch and decided the village couldn't be much farther. They had been hiking for almost six hours. She looked down at her numb feet hidden in the snow. There must be almost as much snow inside my socks as outside my shoes, she thought. Her right foot, in the shoe that had finally lost its sole, was even more benumbed than her left, and she marveled that either one still obeyed her commands to keep walking.

01 December 1943, Wednesday—1600:
Special Air Services Mission, Krushove

They were right on top of the village before they knew it, because the houses lay almost buried in deep drifts. A man they had not seen before ushered them into the first house they came to on the outskirts of town. Walking on a shoveled path between shoulder-high walls of snow, they approached what appeared to be a stable. As they entered a large room, they beat the snow from their clothing. The ten women were led up a flight of stairs into a rough timber hallway and a sizable room, complete with a fireplace and small windows tucked right under the roof. Jens noticed immediately that the windows had glass panes, the fireplace was real, and a blazing fire was sending warmth, unaccompanied by smoke, into the room. The women peeled off as many wet clothes as decently possible, given the lack of privacy that had followed them since leaving Sicily. They placed their soggy shoes and socks near the fire to dry and looked for a place to hang their trench coats so they would be dry enough by bedtime to use as covers.

"The only thing I don't like about getting warm," Jean said, "is that my mercifully numb feet start hurting all over again."

"Did you ever see this much snow in South Dakota, Elna?" Jens asked. "It's almost impossible to make out the buildings—they're nearly buried."

"Yeah," Elna said. "I'm glad we're in a two-story job."

Captain Smith, who had left the party at the door, returned with another man in British uniform and introduced him as Major Palmer. The two men joined them by the fire. After the nurses had answered questions about where they had been and how they had gotten on since crash-landing, the officers explained that they and their companions had been in Albania various lengths of time, up to a year.

"Most of our people parachuted into Greece and walked into Albania," Palmer said. "We're here primarily to help the Albanians harass the Germans and to disrupt Jerry's supply lines and blow up bridges and warehouses whenever possible." Palmer looked and sounded very casual about the main mission of the British in the country.

"Do our people know how many of us are accounted for?" Jens asked.

"Yes," Palmer said. "They've been notified and have already confirmed the message."

"How do you get messages out of here, and where are your headquarters?" Elna asked.

"We have a small wireless that runs on kerosene," Palmer responded. "Our headquarters are in Cairo and we talk to them every night." He smiled. "That is, with Jerry permitting, of course."

"What can the Germans do to stop you?" Tooie asked.

"One way is to try to jam our broadcast so the most Cairo gets is a garbled message," Captain Smith said. "That way, all Cairo knows is that we tried to make contact."

"How much can the Germans learn just by listening in?" Jean asked.

"Not much," Smith said. "All messages are in code, and the code is changed fairly regularly."

"We've already asked Cairo to send some warm socks and underwear for you," Palmer said. "And as soon as we find out how many actually need them, we'll send out an order for shoes."

"Great!" Tooie said. "We can write our sizes down for you."

The two men burst into howling laughter. "I'm afraid we won't be able to accommodate your personal sizes," Palmer said, recovering. He wiped tears from his eyes with the back of his hand. "The shoes will be all men's GI issue in whatever sizes they happen to have on hand." He grinned. "Let's just hope they have some to send us."

"In the meantime," Smith said, "we shall have all the better shoes repaired, just in case we only get a few new pairs." He glanced from person to person. "Repairs take a while here, so in the morning, have your shoes ready to be picked up."

"You'll be shoeless for a while," Palmer said, "but there's nothing you'll have to go out for."

They exuded such confidence and were so matter of fact that Jens felt sure nothing could go wrong while they were in charge.

The two men left and returned an hour later with bullybeef and some of their rations to share. Everyone agreed that by Albanian standards, the British had provided a banquet.

Before leaving, the men told the nurses that they hoped to receive and send a message that night.

"By the way," Major Palmer said, "if you hear low-flying planes, don't be alarmed. They'll be dropping equipment and bodies." He smiled. "'Bodies' is our quaint way of saying additional personnel. We'll always warn you when we know ours are due. However, I don't believe we'll be getting any tonight." He smiled. "Sleep well. We'll be back in the morning to pick up the shoes for repairs. Others will be dropping in to bring you various things. We'll take the best care of you." He smiled even more warmly. "Good night."

The women claimed their places on the floor and turned their backs toward the fire. No one seemed inclined to talk, and one by one they dropped from drowsiness into sound sleep.

Suddenly Jens thought she heard a plane. She opened her eyes in time to see Ann sit up quickly.

"No, it can't be," Jens said. "They're not expecting any."

Soon others were sitting up, listening. The sound became unmistakable, and almost immediately the planes were right overhead. The nurses sat frozen, staring at each other.

Jens's mind was analyzing information as quickly as she received it. It was a heavy plane, and no aircraft of that size would fly so low over and around the mountains if it didn't have to.

Ann, the most pessimistic in the group, was staring at and through Jens with an expression of sheer terror. "Who is it?" she whispered.

Jean and Jens looked at each other and almost laughed.

"Do you think it's the Germans?" Ann asked pleadingly.

A streak of mischief got the best of Jens and Jean. They nodded knowingly and said, "Who else could it be?"

Ann started whimpering and whining, and for a moment Jens thought she would jump out the window.

"For heavens sake, Ann," Jean said, "how do we know any better than you? At least they flew on without bombing or strafing."

But had they flown away? Jens wondered. The same unmistakable roar was approaching again. Ann blanched a ghastly white, and for a moment Jens was sure she'd pass out right where she was sitting.

"Here they come again," Elna said. "Good gosh! How can they fly so low over these jagged mountains?"

"Maybe they're lost," Tooie said. "They darn well better gain altitude or they'll be down here with us."

The noise faded out and the women sat listening. The silence was almost deafening. One by one they lay back down and pulled their coats over themselves.

Jens wrapped yellow parachute silk, one of the items the British provided, around her head and neck to protect herself from the ever present drafts. In less than thirty minutes, everyone was asleep again.

02 December 1943, Thursday—0715: Krushove

The women awakened with the first signs of daylight. The morning was bright and clear, and the snow sparkled in the first rays of the sun. A man stomped up the stairs, as if to warn the nurses of his approach, and brought in an armload of wood for the fire. Firewood appeared to be abundant here, and Jens wondered if that was because there were more trees nearby, or simply that the British had requested and paid for an ample supply.

A young girl appeared with a pan of lukewarm water and a tray of cornbread. The women splashed water on their hands and faces, and ate the breakfast provided for them.

At 0800 Major Palmer and Captain Smith stopped by to pick up the tattered shoes. They apologized for not having more time, but told the nurses they'd visit with them later.

For the first time in three weeks the group had a relative sense of safety, boosted by the feeling that they were on their way back to their own lines. Walking in all kinds of weather had been exhausting, day after day, but Jens soon realized that sitting idle could be worse. Some individuals grated on one another's nerves in close quarters, and a few were almost blood enemies from earlier arguments over things that would not have mattered back in Sicily.

A little before 1300 Major Palmer called from downstairs, "Hello, up there! Are you all dressed? May we come up?"

"Are we dressed?" Jean called back. "We haven't been undressed since we arrived at this house. Come on up."

Palmer, Smith, and a British lieutenant the nurses hadn't seen before, walked into the room.

"Sorry about that," Captain Smith said. "This was the best house we could get near the edge of town, with an owner not too skittish to keep you."

"Oh, we aren't complaining," Jens said. "Just stating facts. Are our shoes safely in the repair shop?"

"They are," Smith said. "But you must remember that repairs here take a little longer than they do in Allied territory. It will be a day or two before they're ready." Smith stopped and looked at the British lieutenant. "This is Lieutenant Gavin Duffy." He smiled. "Gary to his friends."

Duffy was tall, ramrod straight, with jet back hair, dark eyes, wind-burned skin and a crooked grin; Jens judged him to be about thirty. He spoke in a Yorkshire accent, and she wondered at the difference in speech of these three British officers. She marveled to herself that such a little island as England could have produced such varied dialects among people who couldn't have lived very far apart all their young lives.

"Are you one of the 'bodies' they've been expecting?" Jens asked.

"I'm afraid not," Duffy said. "I've been one of the crowd here for a while." He grinned. "My work takes me away from the Mission quite a bit."

"We were certainly glad to have him here last night," Palmer said. "We received word too late to warn you, but we got a rather large drop."

"So that was one of your planes," Jean said.

"I was about to ask if you'd heard it," Palmer said.

"'Heard it!'" Jean exclaimed. "They rolled the wheels on the roof! We almost lost one girl to a heart attack." She leaned toward Palmer. "And while we're on the subject, what in the world was he doing, flying so low between these mountains?"

"He has to fly among the mountains to make his pass," Smith said. "In fact, the drop zone is so short, they can't dump it all on one pass; they have to come back for a second and occasionally a third round. Last night we got the word very late, then the message itself had to be decoded, and there was no time to notify you. We had to scramble to get our fire pots lit to mark the drop zone for them." He paused briefly. "I'm sorry if you were frightened."

"Frightened isn't the word for it," Jean said. "We thought we were going to lose Ann for sure when he came around for his second pass. I was afraid he'd found the place and was possibly coming back to plant a bomb or two."

"It's unfortunate that we couldn't have let you know the plane was ours," Smith said. "As it was, it took us most of the night to pick up all the supplies. Each chute has a pretty fair load on it, and they sink right into this deep snow." He grinned. "But when a chute doesn't open—which happens occasionally, as it did last night—it either buries itself really deep or bursts apart on impact, scattering the contents all over the place."

"Don't things get broken?" Elna asked. "Presuming some of the things you get are breakable." She looked questioningly at the three men. "What kind of supplies do you get in these drops, any-way?"

The three men laughed.

"On one drop," Lieutenant Duffy said, "a tin of milk from a broken pack flew up into a tree, and as we were picking up packages under the tree, we couldn't understand how we were getting our backs splattered with milk of all things. In the daylight we finally saw the tin, way up in the tree, punctured and hanging from a limb."

Everyone laughed. Duffy's story had provided comic relief in the midst of war.

"How did you happen to come to Albania in the first place?" Tooie asked.

"Each of us volunteered for a special group that would work behind enemy lines," Palmer said. "We were trained in demolition and parachute jumping at a location in Africa before we were dropped into Greece. After harassing the Germans in Greece for a while, each of us walked into Albania. As we said, our main mission here is to harass Jerry and help the partisans do the same."

"How did you get past the border checkpoints?" Jens asked.

"We watched the guards for a while, long enough to make an educated guess as to which ones we might be able to pay off. Then we did exactly that," Smith said.

"That sounds pretty risky," Elna said. "How do you know the ones you paid off won't turn around and sell you out to the Germans?"

"We don't!" Palmer said. "We have to trust our training and instinct."

"Just like the pilots who make your supply drops," Jens said. "That sounded like a very heavy plane last night, or was it because it was so low?"

"Both. They use the Wellington bomber," Palmer said.

"A four-engine plane?" Jens asked. "In here?"

"Yes, it's a big one," Palmer agreed. "I can't say how they do it, and frankly, I'm glad to be picking up supplies on the ground rather than dropping them."

They got up, saying they had to check and store their wares and then get some sleep. "Just thought we ought to advise you that the bird last night was a 'friendly,'" Palmer said. They bounced down the steps as though they had slept all night.

Later in the day, the pilots stopped by; they still had shoes, so they could get out and walk. They told the nurses that Palmer and Smith had invited them to go out some night to help blow up a bridge or a warehouse.

"A warehouse!" Tooie said. She looked absolutely incredulous. "Are the Germans and their supplies that close?"

"They're in Korcë," Baggs said. "And that's about ten miles or so from here."

"Yikes! And they drop supplies and keep them that close to the Krauts," Jens said. Her eyes were opened wide, and she sounded shocked.

"As Smith said, this place isn't exactly accessible," Thrasher said, "especially during this time of the year."

"Will you go out with them?" Jean asked. The pilots' response was noncommittal, and Jens decided that they wouldn't.

"Do you know if they have any plans for us in the next couple of days?" she asked.

"If they do, they sure haven't told us," Baggs said. "I think it depends a lot on how fast they receive shoes, socks, and medicines for us."

"That's right," Elna said. "We do need a few things to make us travelworthy again."

The pilots left, assuring the nurses they'd let them know any news as soon as they heard it.

An hour later the downstairs door opened again, and they could hear a man speaking in Albanian. All eyes turned to the stairs as he walked up with a skinned animal on his shoulder. He nodded to the women, laid the animal on the floor near the windows, and announced, "Sheep." Before anyone could say a word, he had started down the steps.

"Look, gals, supper has arrived," Lois announced. "I'll bet it was walking about an hour ago. All we have to do is cut it up and cook it."

They gathered to inspect the carcass and found a large knife laid across its midsection.

"Too bad he didn't bring a pot large enough to cook it whole," Jens said. She picked up the knife and tried to cut into the animal. "This knife is a dull as a round rock!"

"I have a pocket knife," Jean said. "It has to be sharper than that thing."

The women who had pocket knives in their musette bags got them out and began hacking at the sheep. They managed to cut off a hind quarter, but there was no pot large enough to hold even that.

As they were pondering what to do next, three of their sergeants and a very blond curly-haired British soldier walked into the room. Sergeant J.W. Bell introduced himself as "Blondie" and said he was Lieutenant Duffy's wireless operator. The four men moved closer and as they assessed the situation, began laughing and offering all manner of suggestions, none of which was helpful. When the laughter died down, they searched their pockets, and came up with two pocket knives to contribute to the effort.

"Why not roast it whole?" Blondie suggested.

The men examined the fireplace, but couldn't come up with a way to do it.

"All we can do is hack it into pieces small enough to fit into the largest pot we have," Jens said. She held up the pot. "As you can see, it's barely large enough to cook a medium-sized head of cabbage."

"You'll never cook enough in that for all of you," Blondie said. "I'll go downstairs and see if I can find a bigger pot."

"Great!" Tooie said. "We could cook enough for everybody if we had a large enough kettle."

He returned with a bigger container but looked somewhat embarrassed as he handed it over. "It's larger," Blondie said, "but it has a hole in it."

Jens and Tooie inspected the kettle and found that the hole was near the top. "If we put water no higher than the hole, and tilt it away from the hole when we put it on the fire, the meat could cook evenly."

"Okay," Jean said. "Let's try it."

They put the meat in the kettle and the kettle on the fire. The water evaporated rapidly over the hot fire, so they had to keep adding more to the pot. By the time the water was boiling, the meat was burning. Jens used the fork from her mess kit to turn the meat. She hoped her difficulty in getting the tines of the fork into the ever shrinking meat was due to the dullness of the fork rather than the toughness of their dinner.

"It will take all night to cook enough meat for everybody like this."

One of the sergeants had another idea. "I think we could save time if we take some meat back with us and get someone in the house where we're staying to cook it!" They cut off the meat they needed and carried it back to the rest of the men.

02 December 1943, Thursday—1930: Bari, Italy

Captain Lloyd G. Smith was on the sixth floor of the OSS Advance Headquarters building in Bari, preparing for his trip to Brindisi the next morning. It would be the first leg of a long journey to return the Americans safely to their own lines.

Suddenly there was the unmistakable sound of bombs exploding close by. Smith turned off the lights, opened the blackout curtains, and looked out the window to see large, yellowish white flashes and flames climbing high into the sky over the port area that lay three blocks away. A tall building blocked his view of the military ships he knew were anchored in the harbor, but the Luftwaffe was pounding the Port of Bari unmercifully. Flames reached into the air as if to tear the German planes from the night sky. Narrow ribbons of light leaped skyward from search-lights, and tracer bullets left bright trails against the blackness of the sky. A deep thunderous sound exploded into the night, and more fingers of fire clawed at the sky above Bari harbor. Other explosions followed in quick succession.

They've hit a ship, Smith thought. It must have been carrying munitions. The tall building blocking his view of the carnage was outlined in jagged flames that danced against the night and seemed to caress the structure.

Smith pulled the blackout curtains across the window and flipped the light back on in his office. He would have to move quickly to get out of Bari and on the road to Brindisi, where he would board a patrol boat that would take him to the southwest coast of Albania. He would learn later that one of the ships that exploded in the harbor was carrying large quantities of deadly mustard gas, which floated from the port into the city and killed more than one thousand unsuspecting people before it dissipated. He would learn that the only men who knew there was mustard gas aboard that ship were killed when the vessel was bombed. The city that he left on orders from his commanding officer was at the mercy of a death-dealing fog that crept into its streets and homes from the bombed hulk of an American ship. On that night of 2 December 1943, however, Smith's mission was to save lives elsewhere.

02 December 1943, Thursday—2015: Krushove

A little after 2000 hours, the man of the house brought a tray of cornbread to the women. They had just finished eating mutton and drinking what hot broth they had managed to save from the meat and the leaking pot. He left with the hacked up carcass, and the nurses felt sure his family would have a feast on the remaining meat.

"Boy, am I tired," Jens said. "Do you realize that we've been slaving over a hot fireplace for more than five hours? I'm giving up for the night. I shall retire to this nice soft floor, pull my coat over me, and sleep the sleep of the well fed." She wrapped her head in the yellow parachute silk. "This place has the draftiest floor of any place we've stayed so far."

"You know, I need a picture of us in this room so I never forget what it was like," Tooie said. "I wish one of us had brought a camera."

"Not me," Lois said. "I plan to forget the whole thing as soon as we get back."

03 December 1943, Friday—0800: Krushove

It was daylight before Jens heard the other women stirring. No one seemed in a hurry to get up, since they faced another day of idleness.

"How many days have we been here now?" Lois asked.

"This is the third," Jens said. "We arrived here on December 1, so this must be my birthday, December 3."

There was a chorus of "Happy Birthdays!"

"Let's paddle her," Elna suggested.

"I don't have the energy," Tooie said. "Let's wait until some of the men get here to help us."

"Yoo hoo! Are you up?" The British had appeared again at their door.

"Up? You gentlemen have the quaintest questions," Jens said. "Not up off the floor, but awake."

The pilots were with them, and this led the women to expect some important announcement. But the men chatted aimlessly until Lois asked, "Well, what's the news today?"

"We haven't heard anything at all," Captain Smith said. "Baggs, Thrasher, Palmer, and I went to check on shoe repairs earlier. He promised them tomorrow without fail. Some of the men's were ready, so we delivered them and then came here."

"Do you expect any planes tonight?" Jean asked.

"We're always expecting them, sort of, but we have no word yet," Palmer said. "We're hoping to get some 'bodies' tonight, plus some gear for your group."

"Guess what," Tooie said. "It's Jens's birthday today."

"Sweet sixteen, I'm guessing," Smith said. "Has she been soundly spanked yet?"

"Oh, you do that in England too?" Tooie said.

"Do we do that?" Smith asked. "Where do you think you people get all your customs?"

"Oh, come on out of that tree!" Tooie said. "That was ages ago, and if we wanted to be nasty, we could remind you that we won that war."

"Uh, oh! We'll be glad to bury the hatchet," Smith said. "We'll even think up a surprise for Jens."

"I've had as many surprises as I can stand in the past month," Jens said. "I'm always afraid of that final surprise!"

"Don't worry about that," Palmer said. "The Germans can't sneak in that easily. We keep a few people on our payroll to make sure we're aware of Jerry's activities."

"Don't you suppose they do the same?" Jens asked.

"Certainly. Just so they don't start paying ours too," Smith said. "But they'd have to figure out who our guards are, first."

"They must know you're here, what with the planes and all," Jens said.

"Oh, of course they do," Smith said. "I even walked into Korcë one night and looked around." His tone was matter-of-fact.

"You!" Jens exclaimed. "You're rather light-complexioned for that, aren't you?"

"Yes. Well, I was awfully dirty at the time."

Everyone laughed.

"I guess you didn't see any Germans, or vice versa."

"No, fortunately, I didn't. I figured they were all holed up on a cold night."

"Why did you do it? Take such a chance, I mean." Jens was sincerely perplexed.

"Well," Smith said, "after a while, you just have to go and see for yourself. It's like why people climb mountains—because they're there."

"What would the Germans have done if they had caught you?" Jens asked. "I'm guessing you weren't in uniform."

"Actually, I was. I just threw a large Albanian cape over my shoulders. As you know, they reach the knees. I also had boots on." He smiled. "As to the rest of the answer, I try not to think about what Jerry might do if he caught me."

"I'd like to watch a drop some night," Tooie announced.

"I would too," Jens said, "as soon as I get some shoes and can venture forth in the snow. Would it be possible?"

"Sure," Smith said. "We'd be glad to have the company. We'll let you know, if we get word in time. You just have to watch out for the chutes that don't open. You can see the others easily enough."

"How do you see the chutes that don't open?"

"You don't. There's just a thud and then everything in the carton flies every which way."

"I'll think over my rash request," Jens said. "And since I have no shoes, I have a good excuse."

As they got up to leave, Captain Smith said, "We'll hope for planes tonight, but there's no guarantee that they'll come."

It was noon when the men left, and time dragged as the women sat on the floor and watched the fire. In the past weeks, Jens had listened to everyone's life history at least once, knew where each member of the group had been born, where they had gone to school, whether they were married, and if they had their appendices. She and the other women looked forward to visits from the British, not only because they hoped for news about plans for their return to Allied territory but because they enjoyed the stories the men shared about their service behind enemy lines.

About 1700 the British returned in jubilant spirits, carrying a container of ice cream and singing "Happy Birthday" to Jens.

"Where in the world did you get ice cream?" Jens asked.

"We made it," Palmer said. "We begged, borrowed, and bought the ingredients."

"Surely you don't have an ice cream freezer!" Pauleen said.

"No, we haven't," Smith said. "Once we had the ingredients mixed, we dug a hole in a snow bank, put the container in, and swirled it around until we had ice cream."

Jens marveled at soldiers tough enough to blow up bridges and warehouses at night yet gentle enough to go to the very real trouble of making ice cream under such conditions in order to surprise an American nurse on her birthday.

"It's not a cake and candles," Smith said, "but it's the best we could do on such short notice."

"It's absolutely wonderful!" Jens said. "I have never had a more welcome surprise, nor a more thoughtful gift."

The women got their mess kits and helped themselves. After many weeks without sugar of any kind, they reveled in the taste of ice cream, sweet, smooth, and creamy.

"This is a birthday I'll never forget," Jens said.

As the British were leaving, Major Palmer stopped at the head of the stairs. "I'm certain we'll get a message very soon—even to-night, Jerry permitting. In fact, something tells me that tonight we'll finally get the bodies we've been expecting."

The men returned at 2000, shouting for the women to come

with them if they wanted to see a drop. There was a scramble for clothes, and Tooie, Pauleen, and Jean raced down the stairs and out the door to follow them. The rest of the women were still without shoes and waited by the fire, nursing their feet, listening for the planes. They arrived about 2100, flying so low over the house that several of the nurses ducked.

03 December 1943, Friday—2345:
Adriatic Sea, Five Miles from the Albanian Coast

The boat carrying Captain Lloyd G. Smith from Italy to Albania was tossed like a matchbox on the rough sea. The boat's captain was complaining loudly. "We must turn back. If the water is this rough five miles out, landing you safely at Seaview would be impossible."

Eight-foot waves washed across the deck as the small vessel fought its way through a U-turn and headed back to Brindisi. Lloyd Smith hoped the sea would calm by the next night so he could land and start his mission in earnest.

03 December 1943, Friday—2355:
Krushove

Pauleen, Tooie, and Jean returned just before midnight. They took off their coats and sat down heavily to pull off their wet shoes and socks. Lois woke up and asked sleepily, "Any shoes or bodies?"

They were too cold and tired to talk, but the rest of the women speculated and smoked English cigarettes.

"I do hope there are shoes so we can get on our way," Jean said.

"For where?" Jens asked.

"For the coast! Didn't you hear Lieutenant Duffy say earlier today that he had received orders to lead us to the coast for evacuation?" Tooie asked.

"I don't know how I missed that," Jens said. "I must have been in the john. Did he say when?"

"No. We need the shoes, socks, and medicine before we can leave," Jean said.

04 December 1943, Saturday—0815:
Krushove

The nurses awoke in full daylight to find Captain Smith and Lieutenant Duffy sitting by the fire. Beside them were piles of hobnailed shoes and woolen socks that looked as if they would be knee high even on the tallest woman. A second pile contained long johns, scarves, and woolen caps. They were eager for the women to know that they hadn't been forgotten. It seemed almost like Christmas, and only a day after Jens's birthday.

"We've begun planning your actual trip to the coast. Duffy, Blondie, and an interpreter will go with you."

"How far is it and how long will it take us to get there?" Pauleen asked.

Captain Smith smiled. "It depends on how fast you can walk, and whether you run into problems that take you off the planned route."

Suddenly Jens thought of Steffa. They had seen very little of him since the British had arrived on the scene; he didn't seem quite so comfortable with the British as he did with the Americans. Jens thought Steffa might feel glad just to be relieved of the responsibility. She felt pretty sure he would continue with the group as he didn't seem to want to be separated from them.

All the women felt relieved to know they would be heading in the right direction after a nearly a month of just wandering about the country.

05 December 1943, Sunday—2230:
Adriatic Sea, Three Miles off the
Southwest Coast of Albania

The small vessel carrying Captain Lloyd Smith had made it two miles closer to its destination than on 3 December. Smith had encouraged the boat's captain to continue, despite the high, rough seas, but could see that he was losing his determination. They had heard several German patrol boats as they passed along the outer waters in the almost moonless night.

A large wave pushed the boat onto its right side and washed over the pilot's cabin before the vessel righted itself and plunged bow down into the deep trough between two gigantic waves.

"We turn back, Captain," the boat's captain said. "It's worse tonight than it was two nights ago."

The boat made a U-turn and headed back for Brindisi.

"We'll try again in a day or two," Smith said. "This bad weather can't last forever."

07 December 1943, Tuesday—2100: Krushove

Palmer, Smith, and Duffy appeared, looking a bit like Cheshire cats.

"We have good news," Palmer said. The three sat near the fire.

"Great! What is it?" Jens asked.

"You'll start your journey to the coast tomorrow," Smith said. "Duffy will fill you in on a need-to-know basis."

"What time will we leave?" Lois asked.

"Be ready at 0800," Duffy said. "The mules should be packed and ready by then too. One of the mules will carry your belongings; the other two will carry the wireless and the kerosene so we can keep in touch with our headquarters in Cairo—daily, we hope."

"Jerry permitting," Tooie said.

Palmer and Smith laughed. "Exactly!" Smith agreed.

"Be sure you're packed and ready," Duffy said. "It's imperative that we leave as early as possible. Get a good night's sleep. We have a lot of territory to cover tomorrow."

The men left, and the women gathered their few belongings, stuffed them into their musette bags, and turned in before 2200.

07 December 1943, Friday—2330: British Advance Base: Seaview, Southwest Albanian Coast

The boat anchored a half-mile off the coast and put Captain Lloyd Smith ashore by rowboat. He used a switch-back trail and climbed the 800 feet to reach the coastal cave that served as the base headquarters. His orders were to wait there for information from Cairo regarding the location and movements of the American party.

08 December 1943, Wednesday—0010: Krushove

It was just after midnight when Jean asked, "Did you hear that? Planes. I think there are two of them."

They came in low over the roofs of the houses.

"I wonder why they're so late tonight," Tooie said drowsily and drifted back into sleep.

At 0730 Lieutenant Duffy called up the stairs. Waiting at the bottom with him were Major Palmer, Captain Smith, and four tall sergeants wearing the berets of the Cold Stream Guards. Jens couldn't decide who was more surprised, the nurses or the four men.

"Oh, look!" Lois said. "The 'bodies' arrived!" Duffy, Smith, and Palmer stood with wide grins, taking in the scene. With typical British humor they hadn't let on to the four newcomers that ten of the Americans they were getting ready to evacuate were women.

One of them looked at Smith. "How long have they been here, and do they have to leave today?"

They stood and talked for only a few minutes before the mules arrived and they started packing up.

Lieutenant Duffy called the group to assemble around him.

"Before we get started, there are a few things you need to know." Duffy's Yorkshire seemed impersonal, but everyone could tell from his eyes that he was deadly serious and meant his words for each individual in the party. "For starters you'll have to walk five or six hours every day. Now that you have new boots and extra socks, we should be able to do that. We'll gradually increase that time as you and your feet get conditioned to walk farther and faster." His eyes swept across every face. "The pace will be only one difficulty for you. You can expect scanty accommodations, little food, delays in acquiring mules, and the strong possibility of running into Germans. We've hired several Albanian guides to accompany us. In short, this won't be a cakewalk, but if you want to get back to your own lines, you must obey my orders immediately and without question. I'll use all I've learned during my time in this country to get you back, safe and in good condition. I ask, I demand, that you put a full 100 per cent into every day we are together on this journey. If any of you slacks off, all of you will suffer. So—if you want to get back to your own base, do what I tell you, and do it as quickly as possible." He adjusted the sling of his rifle strap across his shoulder. "Any questions?" It sounded more like a challenge than an invitation. No one spoke.

"All right then," Duffy said, "we'll get started immediately."

Those remaining in Krushove said goodbye and wished the group a safe journey.

Once again they had to walk in single file, since there were only narrow paths in the deep snow. Jens felt liberated at being outside again after five days in one room. As they left the village, she stopped and looked back. She had seen only small areas from the windows and now discovered that they were on the summit of a beautiful, snow-covered mountain. An Albanian who was walking behind her pointed to a nearby peak and said, "Albani." He pointed toward a more distant one and said, "Greco," and toward still another to their left and said, "Yugoslavia."

They were at Albania's back door. The trail went abruptly downhill, and the group was soon out of the snow.

9 Lieutenant Duffy Leads the Way

Report of Lieutenant Gavin B. Duffy, SOE, British Military Mission, Albania

[8 December 1943]
Krushove M. 99 to Gjergievice, M. 84

We moved off from Krushove at approximately 0800 hrs in the direction of Voskopoj, M. 96. We arrived at Voskopoj and staged a short halt in order to collect bread and cheese; also to fix up by 'phone five houses at Gjergievice for accommodating the party. The foodstuffs were eventually produced by the "SHTABIT" (Military Commandant). So I pushed on. The journey so far had been only about two hours and travel not so bad, so I increased the pace, and everyone was pleased because it was freezing.

Eventually we arrived at our destination at approximately 15.00 hrs. We gathered together the "Council" (Administration Group) of the village, which was Moslem, who fairly quickly regulated the different groups in their specific houses. I called around the different houses in the course of the evening, and found everybody quite content under the circumstances. It must be remembered that nearly all Moslem villages in ALBANIA, with the exception of two, (these I have never visited), are absolutely ridden with lice, so by the time I paid my respects to the party, these ever present companions were just making their presence felt. Sensing this, I informed every one of our time of departure on the morrow, and beat a hasty retreat.

9 December 1943, Thursday—0800: En Route to Panerit

The group assembled with Gary at 0800, and waited for his signal to start.

"I hope we can do as well as yesterday," Gary said. He made eye contact with each member of the party. "Are we all set?" When no one raised an objection, he strode off and the Americans followed him.

Sergeant Zeiber ran up the line and stopped when he reached Jean, Marky, and Jens.

"Eldridge was real sick and vomited most of the night," Zeiber said.

"Let's have him ride on one of the mules and hope he'll be all right," Jean said. She handed him her coat liner, asked Jens for hers and gave it to him too. "Wrap these around his legs to help him keep warm."

They caught up with Elna, who also was riding.

"How are you feeling?" Jens asked.

"I feel generally lousy. Maybe I've got the grippe," Elna said.

Marky wrapped her liner around Elna's hips and back. "Do you want more on your legs?"

"No, I'm not really chilly. In fact, I think I can walk." She leaped off her mule. "Maybe someone else needs to ride."

She didn't convince anybody but insisted on walking anyway.

About noon they stopped at the village of Panerit for food and rest. Eldridge looked terrible. His face was gray and his body limp. Two of the sergeants carried him into the house.

"How are you doing, Eldridge?" Jens asked, concerned at his appearance.

"Not so good. My stomach ulcer bled on me about two years ago, and this feels pretty much the way it did then," Eldridge said.

"Stomach ulcers? How old are you?" Jens asked.

"Twenty-one."

"Did you vomit blood last night or any dark-colored fluid?" Marky asked.

"I don't know. I was outside in the dark when I threw up."

Everyone would have preferred to keep going, but Jens and Jean suggested to Gary that Eldridge really needed to stop and rest.

"About the most we can do is keep him quiet, but it may be the wisest move for all of us," Jens said. "If he can get some rest, he may be able to travel better."

Gary agreed, and Eldridge was carried to the house where Jens, Marky, Pauleen, and Jean would spend the night. They decided that sleep might be the best thing for Eldridge, so they gave him an injection of morphine and covered him with their coats and liners to keep him warm. They had no milk, so they gave him a little water. He slept through the night.

10 December 1943, Friday—0830: En Route from Panerit

In the morning Eldridge looked much better and said he felt fine. He and everyone else wanted to move on. Elna reported that she too was practically well and could travel without any problems.

They were on the trail again about 0830, but in deference to their convalescents, Gary decided to stop early and spend the night in Costomicka. The villagers told them that enemy troops were all around the area. Jens wondered if "enemy" meant Germans, Ballista, or both.

Report of Lieutenant Gavin B. Duffy, SOE

[10 December 1943]
Panerit, M. 84 to [Costomicka]

The party assembled at 08.00 hrs with the intention of making FRASHERE, M. 73. A slight delay of two hours occurred in producing mules and rather held in abeyance the above destination. Finally I decided to carry on ahead with the walking members of the party, leaving the riders behind

to wait for mules. Myself, with my complement, reached the
valley where the River Ossum [Osum] runs through. At this
time of the year, the river was quite high and impossible to
wade across. I removed two horses from a nearby field,
placing two members of the party on each horse, which were
led by the locals who volunteered after slight persuasion.
After one hour and a half, we did succeed in getting all the
party across. By this time it was becoming dark and cold so I
decided to make for COSTOMICKA, which we reached
after a solid hour's climbing. Accommodation here was
splendid, lice in the minority. The people of the village
(L.N.C.) were, however, very much afraid of a reprisal by a
BALLI force who were in a village one hour away. At this
time the L.N.C. forces in KORCA area were carrying out
specialized recruiting campaigns, that is to say that Riza
KOHELI, L.N.C. Battalion Commander, who in the past
week had removed from a BALLI village over 1,000 sheep.
GERMANS in their country, fighting for liberty, and these
two parties carry out a lease and lend project!

[11 December 1943]
Costomicka to Malinj
   I had intended to make for Krashove this day, but was
thwarted by a report of a BALLI concentration at the above
place. My interpreter refused to accompany me to the said
BALLI village. To travel at this stage without an ENGLISH
speaking ALBANIAN, threatened to be no fun, therefore, I
had to change en route my original destination, passing
through a large number of partisans who had taken up
position on the hills opposite where the BALLI forces were
gathered. Sensing a clash, I pushed the party ahead, making a
slight detour and arrived at MALINJ.
   We had, during the course of this day, heard persistent
rumours of an Allied invasion at VALONA [Vlorë] and
DURAZZO [Durrës]. This rumour did not affect the party
as a whole, but did incline to make the two pilots slightly
light-headed. They did think their walking days were over. I

immediately rebuked them severely, pointing out that they, like myself, were part of an organized force, namely, the English and American army and not party to a rabble they had experienced in this country. I pointed out that this was the seventh time I heard of the Allies landing, but would that night signal to my HQ for confirmation and any change in plans. Copy of message sent that night—"No. 2/11/12. Have heard persistent rumours of invasion stop YANKS wish to hear as soon as possible any change in previous plans."

Answer to this signal received the next day at ODRICAN to the effect that it was just a rumour and to carry on as previously arranged.

[12 December 1943]
MALINJ to ODRICAN M. 68

This day was indeed filthy weather, rain, mud, and very cold. Therefore, not to cause any delay in accommodation, I left one hour before the party for ODRICAN. When the party did arrive, they did indeed receive a grand reception from the village (Christian).

Good houses had been selected by the Council and the members of the party quickly dispersed to the different homes.

This short journey of four hours that day suited me perfectly, as I wished the batteries to be charged and also await confirmation of the invasion. My signal that night was as to my position and also warning TILMAN of my E.T.A. PREMET [Përmet], M. 62.

12 December 1943, Sunday—1245: Seaview, British Advance Base, Southwest Coast

Captain Lloyd G. Smith, OSS, had waited in the coastal cave since his arrival on Tuesday for word concerning the American party.

Commander Glen, British Naval Liaison Officer at the base, informed him that Major Tilman was in Kuc and might have information regarding the American group. The captain obtained a Ballist guide, a shepherd by occupation, and started toward Kuc at a slow and deliberate pace.

Report of Captain Lloyd G. Smith, OSS, to Colonel West, OSS

13 December 1943

On December 13, 1943, I arrived at Dukati at 1200 hours, and was met there by about fifty armed Ballista who tried to persuade me not to enter the Partisan territory, which was necessary in order to get to Kuc. In this area the dividing line between LNC and Ballist territory was the pass between DUKATI and TERBACI. After an hour's discussion, during which my guide became scared and wanted to go back, it was decided that since I was going, despite the warning of the Ballists, they would give me three guides to take along with the provision that I would bring them back to Ballist territory. In the days prior to my arrival at Dukati, the Partisans then in TERBACI, had had a fight with the people of DUKATI. In this fighting, over 30 people had been killed or wounded. I also received information in DUKATI that the Germans were expected to be in TERBACI.

I left for TERBACI at 1330 hours, and met 30 Partisans coming up the TERBACI side of the pass at approximately 1545 hours. They were armed with 8 light machine guns (Breda 30's). Some were carrying both English and Italian made grenades. Several different makes and calibers of rifles were carried but, for the most part, these were of Italian manufacture. One of the Partisans accompanied us to TERBACI where we arrived at 1750 hours.

In Terbaci we were taken to a house where there was a girl interpreter. They all seemed to be very glad to see me, but showed disappointment that I was accompanied by three Ballist guides. They also embarrassed me by asking why the Allies were not making good progress in northern Italy. They were very quick to point out how well the Russians were doing on their front. Here also for the first time, they wanted to take my three Bals, prisoners. I told them that I had guaranteed the safety of my guides, and would go no where without them, that if I could not depart, my mission could not be completed, and that when my government asked me why it had not been completed, I would be obliged to state that the Partisans would not allow me to proceed.

The girl interpreter suggested that I go and see the Commandant of the Vth Partisan Brigade whose headquarters were at Ramishti. I accordingly started for Ramishti, neatly placed in the center of a squad of ten Partisans. The Commandant met me about an hour from Ramishti and insisted that I ride his horse the remainder of the way. We arrived at the Commandant's headquarters at 2400 hours. Since the Commandant was very busy and had to go back out to see after his men, I had to get what information I could from the Commissar through the girl interpreter. They all tried to get me involved in political discussions at various times.

Report of Lieutenant Gavin B. Duffy, SOE

[13 December 1943]: Odrican to Premet [Përmet], M. 62

I left the party from ODRICAN for six hours trek to PREMET; this turned out to be eight hours. We arrived at the outskirts of PREMET after walking down the main highway to BERAT for two hours. How that party walked down that highway! A bridge used to link the highway across the river VIOSO [Vjose] into the town of PREMET. As the GERMANS had a week previously entered PREMET and burnt a large proportion of the remaining houses, it was found necessary to destroy this bridge and put in its place a sort of swinging suspension. It would take unloaded mules and pedestrians. On the other side, all the party, plus luggage etc., boarded a big WOP Diesel truck and drove into the town amidst crowds of cheering people. Here good accommodation was arranged and I sent a letter to Major TILMAN warning him of our arrival the next day at SHEPR.

14 December 1943, Tuesday—0815:
En Route from Përmet to Shepr

The group assembled and waited for Gary. After fifteen minutes of standing in the cold, several of the party began to ask questions.

"Has anyone seen Gary or Blondie this morning?" Jens asked.

"I saw them about a half hour ago, and they were both working on the radio," Steffa said.

"Well, then what's the idea of rushing us outside?" Jens complained. "I would think we'd be less conspicuous and a little warmer inside."

"I think getting us outside as soon as possible was the villagers' idea," Baggs said. "The people in the house where I stayed told us that the Germans use this road fairly frequently for motorcycles and cars. They said they felt very unsafe with us around." He shrugged. "I can't say that I blame them, what with the Krauts burning some of their villages."

Everyone in the group understood, but understanding gave no protection against the freezing temperatures. They paced, stamped their feet, and jumped up and down to fight the numbing effects of the cold.

At 0920 Gary appeared and informed the group of the plans for the day.

"When you get down on the road, don't bunch up. Spread out four or five to a group and move along at a fast walk until you cross the bridge," Gary said.

Blondie and two sergeants took off ahead of the party. It was very open country with the first intact bridge the group had seen since Berat. The road curved around a ridge, so it was impossible to see anyone or anything approaching. Jens found herself listening for motorcycles.

Farther down the road Jens saw one of the guides standing in the brush to the left of the bridge, motioning for them to come toward him. Suddenly two men stepped out of the bushes just ahead of Gary.

Jens's heart stood still as she checked each side of the road for a place to dive into quickly. She was relieved when she saw Gary and Panda, his interpreter, walk directly toward the men. The group stopped in their tracks and watched. In a second Jens realized that Gary knew the two and was giving them both unadulterated hell. With his hands on his hips, he looked at Panda to translate for him. Jens felt sure that after Gary had called them every kind of SOB, Panda in his slow and polite way, had said something to the effect of, "My dear gentlemen, you have distressed Mr. Gary no end." At least the tone of his voice, the earnest conversation he had with them, and the expressions on their faces led her to that conclusion. But his gentleness only seemed to make Gary more angry. His face was a deep shade of red as he motioned the party forward with a quick movement of his arm. The two men ran along with everyone else, and it was Jens's best guess that they had been sent out earlier to scout the trail but hadn't made it back before Gary finally gave up and started out.

The ground was flat and boggy, making it difficult to keep up the pace that was being set. They slowed as they caught up with the group that was ahead of them. The Vjose River was wide and swift as it came around the curve and meandered its way along their route. Jens spotted some of their gang riding in a flat-bottomed boat across the river. As the boat returned from the far side, she could see that it was wider and shallower than most American rowboats. It was hauled back and forth across the river by men on both shores who pulled on ropes attached to each end of the small craft. Another man stood in the rear of the boat, pushing and steering it with a long pole.

In just a few trips the entire party was transported across the swiftly moving water. They were again in wide open land, and Gary was in a hurry to get them out of it. Jens and her companions had to run to catch up with the rest.

Conversation picked up after they had hiked for almost two hours.

"Whatever happened to the American OSS man who was supposed to meet us?" Jens asked.

"Gary said he's in the country," Baggs answered. "He landed a couple of days ago."

"Really? Well, where is he?" Tooie asked.

They hurried to catch up to Gary. Jens hoped he'd share information, since they already knew something about the subject. Tooie stopped directly in front of Gary so she had to look up at him. "Was an American really put ashore? Baggs says he's coming to meet us. How will he know which trail to take?"

Gary smiled. "I'm sure he is equipped to keep track of us. He's in the country all right—Captain Smith is his name. The last report said he'd started walking toward us with two guides, but he's been unheard of since."

"When did he arrive?" Tooie asked.

"As far as I could make out, he was put ashore in the early morning hours of the tenth."

"Good heavens! He must be on the wrong trail," Tooie said.

"He'll find us," Gary said.

"Captain Smith," Jens said. "Do you know if that's his real name? We wondered the same about your Captain Smith, you know."

Gary looked straight at Jens and shrugged. "We don't need aliases for this business. The Germans don't care what our real names are when they shoot us."

"Well, I sure hope he's all right," Tooie said.

Gary had suddenly become more talkative, but not at all cheerful. "If they got proper guides for him, he's all right. But if he was expected, it's easy to walk into a trap in this game."

Report of Gavin B. Duffy, SOE

[13 December 1943]: Premet [Përmet], m.62 to Shepr, M.61
If one follows the map of the distance between these two points it indicates just about one inch. In actual fact it took almost seven hours of what I consider the worst climbing in ALBANIA, which is over the top of Mt. Nermerska 1,846 metres. This was the second mountain of this type the AMERICANS had climbed. The remarks of some nurses longing for the plains of their own country were really amusing.

Report of Captain Lloyd G. Smith, OSS

14 December 1943
On the morning of December 14, 1943, the Commandant

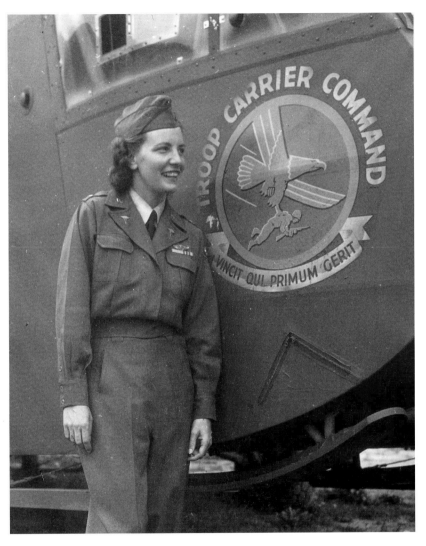

Lieutenant Agnes Jensen, 1944.

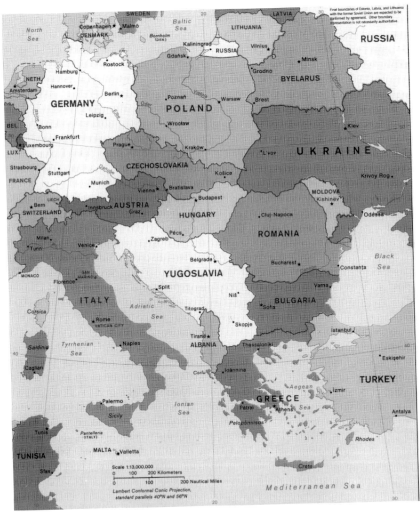

Bordering Yugoslavia and Greece, Albania is just across the Adriatic Sea from Italy. Bari, the planned destination for the flight, is located just above the Italian heel. Courtesy of the National Technical Information Service, U.S. Government, Springfield, Virginia.

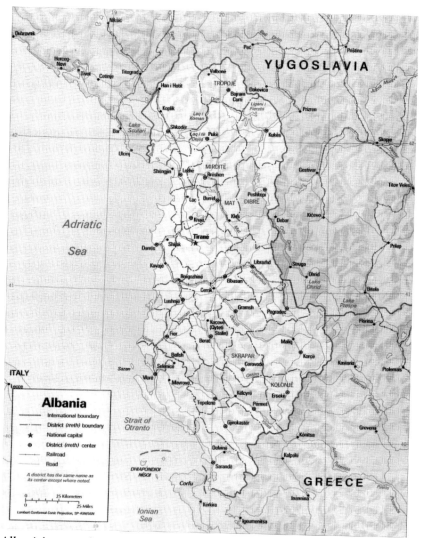

Albania's rugged mountains were a major obstacle in the nurses' escape to
Allied lines. Courtesy of the National Technical Information Service, U.S.
Government, Springfield, Virginia.

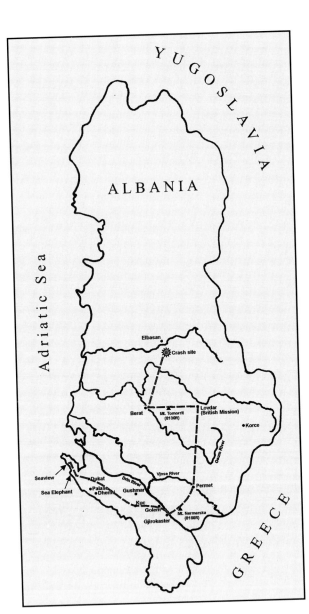

Albanian Villages, Cities, and River Crossings along
Escape Route, 1943-1944

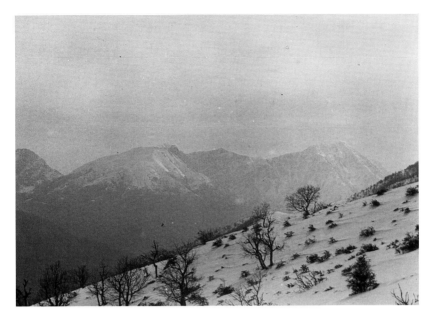

In this view of the Albanian terrain from the east side of the "last mountain," the widest and deepest "V" is the Dukat-Terbaci pass, dividing line between the partisans and Ballists. Courtesy of Lt. Col. Lloyd G. Smith, AUS (Ret.).

(Map at left) Many of the towns and villages visited were very small, with only a few houses, and they are too numerous to note on this map. They are listed here in the order of the party's escape route and lie between the cities and locations marked with asterisks, which do appear on the map.

Crash site south of Elbasan*
Pashtrani
Berat*
Matishave
Bargulla
Dobrusha
Derzhezha
Leshnija
Mt. Tomorrit* (alt. 8136 ft.)
Terlioria
Lovdar*
Krushove
Gjergievice
Panerit
Osum River*
Gostomicka/Costomicka
    [spelling used interchangeably]
Malinj
Odrican
Permet on the Vjose River*

Mt. Nermerska* (alt. 8186 ft.)
Shepr
Gjirokastër*
Mashkulon
Zhulat
Progonat
Golem*
Kalonja
Karla
Doksat
Saraginishte
Drin River*
Midhar
Golem*
Kuc*
Kalarat
Terbaci
Dukat*
Seaview*
Sea Elephant*

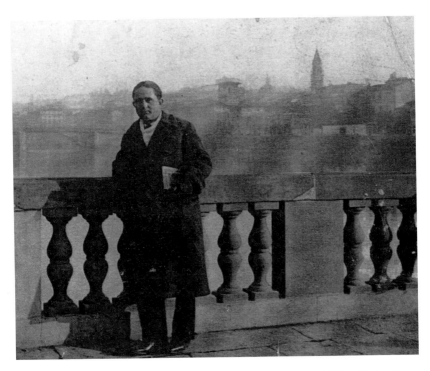

(Above) Kostig Steffa as a student in Italy prior to World War II. Author's archives. *(Below)* Lieutenant Gavin (Gary) Duffy, SOE, led the stranded nurses, medics, and flight crew from Krushove to the coast during the escape from Nazi-occupied Albania. British Army Photograph.

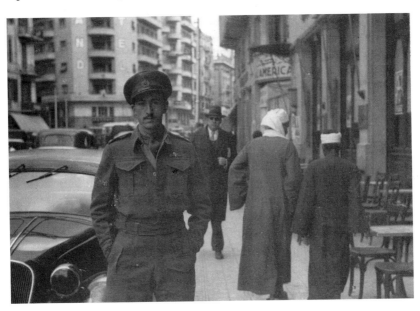

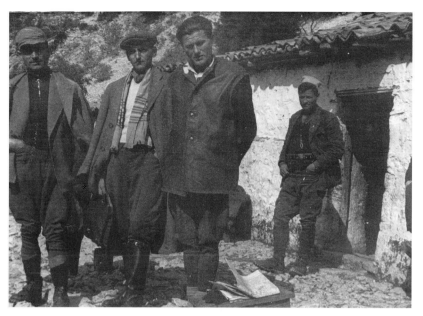

Hodo Meto (without hat) and his cousin (second from left) helped Major Smith rescue the last three flight nurses of the 807th Evacuation Squadron, March 1944. Courtesy of Lt. Col. Lloyd G. Smith, AUS (Ret.).

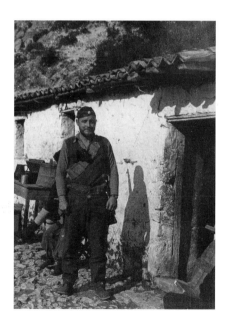

Major Lloyd Smith, OSS, in Albania to evacuate the last three nurses, March 1944. Courtesy of Lt. Col. Lloyd G. Smith, AUS (Ret.).

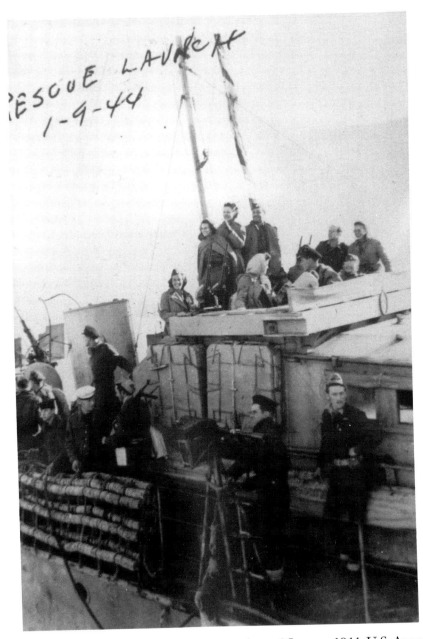

The nurses' rescue boat arrived at Bari, Italy, on 9 January 1944. U.S. Army Photograph.

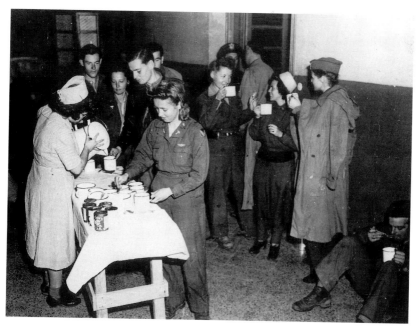

(Above) Members of the 807th Flight Evacuation Squadron were welcomed with hot coffee on their return to Bari. U.S. Army Photograph. *(Below)* Seven of the thirteen flight nurses of the 807th Evacuation Squadron after returning from Albania. From left to right, Lois Watson, Lillian Tacina, Pauleen Kanable, Elna Schwant, Ann Kopsco, Frances Nelson, and Ann Markowitz. Author's archives.

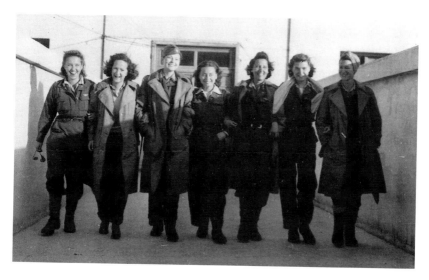

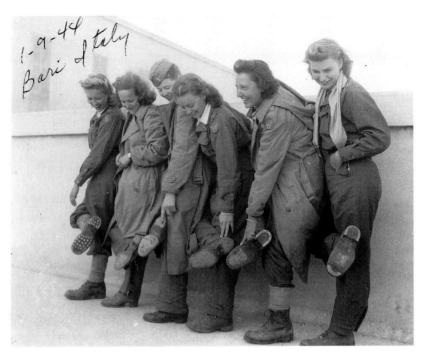

After an 800-mile trek out of Nazi-occupied Albania, the nurses' Army-issue boots were well beyond being broken in. From left to right, Lois Watson, Lillian Tacina, Pauleen Kanable, Elna Schwant, Ann Kopsco, and Frances Nelson. Author's archives.

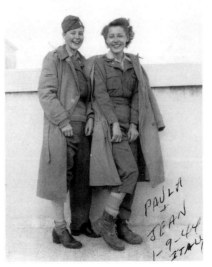

Lieutenants Pauleen Kanable and Jean Rutkowski the day of their return from Albania. Author's archives.

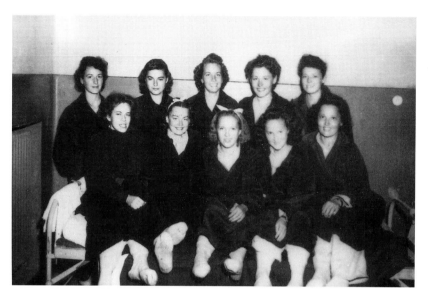

(Above) The army flight nurses during their hospitalization following their return to Bari, Italy. Front, from left to right: Gertrude "Tooie" Dawson, Elna Schwant, Lois Watson, Lillian Tacina, and Ann Kopsco. Back, from left to right: Ann Markowitz, Frances Nelson, Agnes "Jens" Jensen, Jean Rutkowski, and Pauleen Kanable. Author's archives. *(Below)* Gertrude "Tooie" Dawson and Agnes "Jens" Jensen (standing) in the Twenty-sixth General Hospital in Bari. Author's archives.

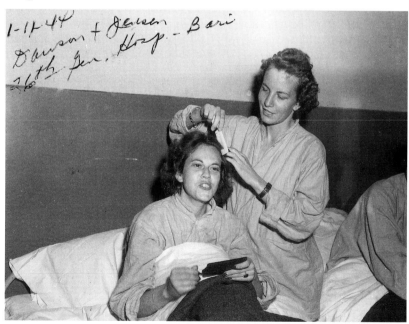

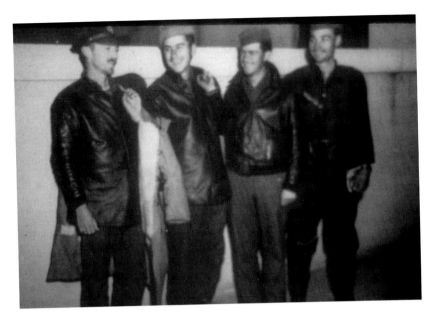

(Above) The four-man flight crew of the ill-fated air evacuation flight, Lieutenants James Baggs and Charles Thrasher and Sergeants Richard Lebo and Willis Shumway. Author's archives. *(Below)* Technical sergeants of the 807th Evacuation Squadron at the Twenty-sixth General Hospital in Bari. The soldier in bed is Sergeant James P. Cruise. Author's archives.

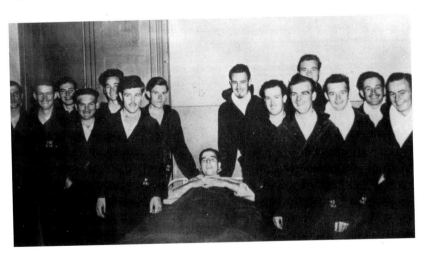

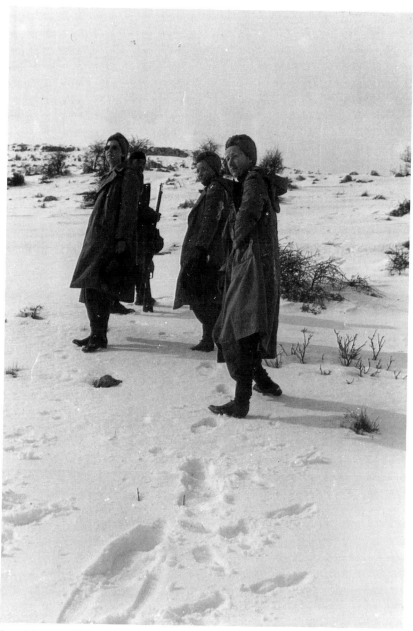

Ann Maness, Wilma Lytle, and Helen Porter in the snowcapped mountains of Albania in March of 1944. Courtesy of Lt. Col. Lloyd G. Smith, AUS (Ret.).

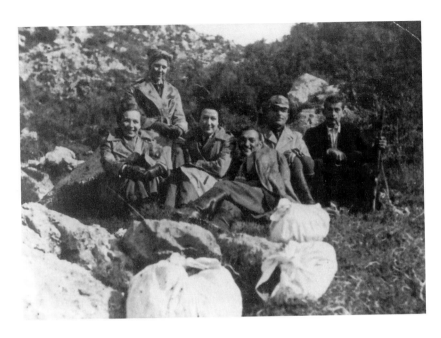

(Above) Left to right: Wilma Lytle, Helen Porter, Ann Maness, and Albanian guides. *(Below)* Ann Maness, an Albanian partisan, and Wilma Lytle on their hike out of Albania. Courtesy of Lt. Col. Lloyd G. Smith, AUS (Ret.).

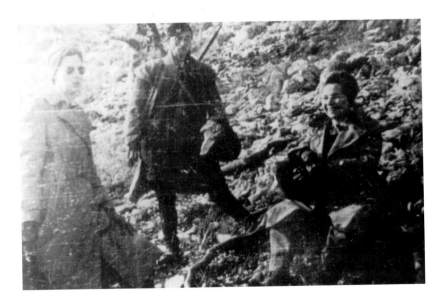

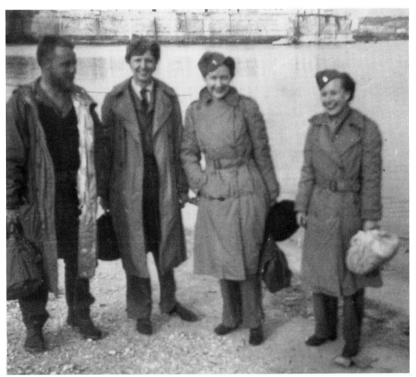

Major Lloyd G. Smith (left) with Ann Maness, Helen Porter, and Wilma Lytle in Otranto, Italy, March 1944. Courtesy of Lt. Col. Lloyd G. Smith, AUS (Ret.).

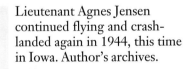

Lieutenant Agnes Jensen continued flying and crash-landed again in 1944, this time in Iowa. Author's archives.

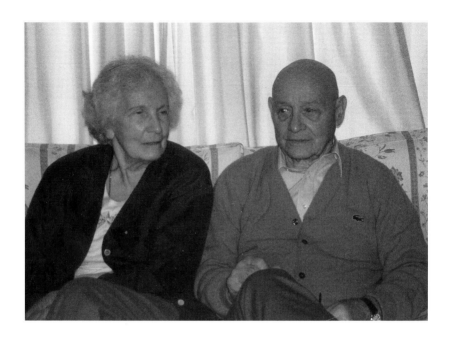

Agnes Jensen Mangerich and Lloyd G. Smith, October 1997. Author's archives.

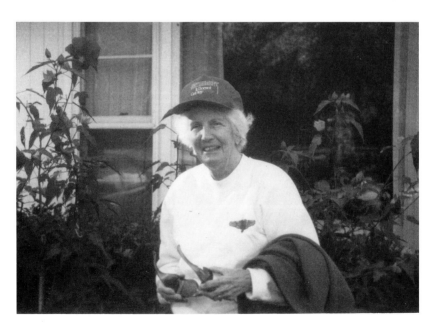

had not yet returned. However at about 0900 hours, an English demolition sergeant (one of Major Tilman's men) came in. He told me that Major Tilman had gone back to Shepr. The sergeant had no information on the American Party. At this time the Commissar said that he would send out scouts to secure information, and that I could see him in Kuc in about ten days. I then decided that since Tilman was not in Kuc, that I could go back to the Base and see if any information had come by W/T.

I left Ramishti at 1200 hours and started back to Terbaci accompanied only by my original three Ballist guides. The night before, the Commandant had told me that the guides could travel safely with me wherever I wanted to go. On arrival at Terbaci at 1500 hours, I was told immediately that the Germans and the Partisans were fighting in the Pass. Since the Pass was blocked and I did not want to start over the mountain either to the north or to the south of the pass at such a late hour, I decided to wait until the next morning; possibly by that time the Germans would be out of the Pass. If I could get an early start, I could cross the mountain either to the north or the south.

This same evening, I noticed Partisans coming back down from the Pass with German boots, seven K98Ks (the German standard army rifle) and one machine gun #34, and three PO8s (Luegers). I estimated that at least ten Germans must have been killed, to secure this quantity of arms and equipment. Every Partisan I met, claimed he alone had killed from eight to ten Germans.

10 Germans Strike Again

Report of Captain Lloyd G. Smith, OSS

[15 December 1943]

The next morning (Dec. 15, 1943) at 0730 hours, I was awakened by a messenger from the Commissar informing me that the three Ballist guides had been taken prisoners and that he would not allow them to accompany me. I went down to his headquarters and had a long argument after which it was agreed that the men would be released to me but that I would not be allowed to proceed to Dukati with them until he got a note of clearance from the Commandant.

At this time I noticed that the villagers were getting very nervous and jittery. At about 1500 hours I heard firing (rifle) from the direction of Barataj. The Commissar came in and told me that the Germans were coming and that I could leave immediately with my three Bal guides but that I could not go through the pass since the Germans were still there.

I left Terbaci at 1630 hours and after climbing over a snow-covered, two thousand meter high mountain I arrived at a house on the outskirts of Dukati at 0500 hours, December 16, 1943. From this point a guide was sent on ahead to find an English-speaking friend of mine. The guide returned with my friend and I was informed that there were thirty Germans in the village. He told me that they could get me through the town with very little trouble. Dressed in a shepherd's hat and long, native coat, I walked through the center of the village, past a squad of Germans who had their rifles stacked and climbed into a truck and rode down the highway to about one kilometer from the point where the trail goes over the mountain to the coastal base.

After getting out of the truck I went on the trail to the right of the road until the truck had disappeared. I then recrossed the road and went to a house belonging to a good friend of the personnel at the Base at 1700 hours.

15 December 1943, Wednesday—0840: En Route to Maskulon

From Shepr they started out much the same as other mornings, two or three people riding mules, the rest walking. It was extremely cold, and many walked with their heads down to keep the biting wind out of their faces and to make breathing a little easier. Every now and then someone would look up quickly to make sure they were following the people who were following the guides. They climbed up and down the countryside for hours. As they came down the side of the last ridge, a wide grassy field spread out in front of them.

"This is like walking on air after the rocky terrain we've been through," Jens said. "Thank goodness for the repaired shoes and extra socks." She followed several sergeants across the green field. As she got closer to them, she heard their conversation.

"They could easily land a C-47 here, couldn't they, Lieutenant Baggs?" Sergeant Owen asked.

"Yeah, easy!" Baggs answered.

"This is the only other place in the whole country that I've seen that's large enough to land a plane of any kind," Jens said.

Steffa had caught up with them and overheard the discussion. "It used to be an Italian airfield," Steffa said. "So far the Germans haven't used it."

Two young Albanians with dark, ragged capes flapping around them came trotting to meet them. They talked to Panda and pointed, and in a matter of seconds Gary said, "It's getting dark, so instead of going on, as planned, we'll stay in Gjirokastër for the night." He motioned in the direction they were to go. The party stumbled up a slope to a wide, rough gravel road. As they walked along the edge, Gary urged them into a dogtrot. Then the climb toward the city continued along cobblestone steps that no vehicle, Jens felt sure, could negotiate.

When they reached the top, they were led into a pitch-dark building. They waited until someone with a small kerosene or oil lamp showed them the way to a room where a couple of dim light bulbs hung from the ceiling. It was a school room, a primary school, Jens guessed from the small desks they tried to occupy. Gary sat down at a table in the front of the room with several townspeople around him. Panda must have moved quickly to the heart of the matter, for in less than ten minutes they were following their hosts to their homes, which were mercifully close by.

The house in which Jens stayed was much more comfortable than any they had been lodged in so far, and for a change she could even sit in a chair with her feet hanging down. Jens was happy to see a young girl of the house appear with a bowl of eggs and a huge, heavy iron skillet—until she put big spoonfuls of heavy grease into the pan and broke the eggs into it. They just swam around in the fat, which stuck to the eggs when the Americans tried to eat them later. Jens would have passed up this greasy offering, as hungry as she was, except that the family sat and watched them eat.

Fats had begun to nauseate her, at times causing such abdominal cramps and pressure under her diaphragm that she feared she had an inflamed gall bladder. Now she felt so tired and sick that she wanted only to try to go to sleep.

They were led to a room where a large feather tick was rolled out on the floor. The hostess and her daughter helped them undress. Jens was sure they wanted to check their clothes for lice. She lay down and hoped her nausea would pass and thanked God for shelter with an inside toilet.

16 December 1943, Thursday—0915: En Route to Zhulat

The group walked down the trail silently. The air turned suddenly colder as the sun disappeared behind a large cloud. Jens walked with her head down to keep the icy wind from her face.

Around 1430, she bumped into some of the men on the trail, and looking up, she saw a stranger talking to Panda and Steffa. She moved up closer to hear what was being translated, then saw smoke on the trail ahead. She peered through and around the smoke and saw stacks of charred stones and smoldering poles. In an instant, she realized that the ruins before them must be Maskulon, the village that had been their original destination the previous night.

Lois joined Jens at the front of the line. "Imagine if we had gotten here about nine o'clock last night!"

From the tone of the men's voices, the news was disastrous. Jens turned to Steffa. "Translate for us, Steffa. What are they saying?"

"This man says the Germans came yesterday. They took blankets, food, five chickens, and two goats. After chasing the people out of their houses on the pretext of a search, they set fire to the houses from the inside. Many of the villagers ran off to hide," he said, "because they were afraid some might be taken as captives."

Gary questioned the villagers through the interpreters. "Did the Germans have any reason that you know of for reprisals? Have you seen much of the Germans or their activities before this?"

One distraught villager talked on and on until Steffa patted his arm gently and stopped his flow of words. "He says he doesn't know why they raided his village, but even if they took everything, why did they have to burn the houses? Now they have no place to live, and winter is here."

Gary wanted more information. "Have they burned any other villages that you know of?"

The man shook his head, said a few more words, and waited for Steffa to translate.

"He says they heard of some Germans here lately, but this was totally unexpected and unexplainable, since there are no active partisans here."

"Ask him how far the next village is," Jens said.

"About four hours, maybe a little more," Panda said.

Jens looked at Gary. "This is the village we were supposed to stay at last night?"

Gary wrinkled his nose and scratched his head. "Yeah, as a matter of fact, it is." He looked over the smoldering ruins and spoke more to himself than to anyone else. "Now wouldn't that have been a mess!"

Gary was tight-lipped as he led the way toward the next village. They arrived at Zhulat in just over three and a half hours and waited to be assigned to individual houses. Before they split up, Jens asked several of her companions, "Where are the two British?"

"I think they've already gotten into a house by themselves," Baggs said. "Gary wanted to get word out about the Germans burning the village and was afraid it would take all night."

"He certainly has become an intense person," Tooie said. "I wish he'd relax a little."

"His job wasn't designed for relaxing," Baggs said. "How old do you think he is?"

"About thirty or thirty-two," Jens guessed.

Baggs smiled. "He's twenty-two!"

"He's younger than most of us!" Jens exclaimed.

"Yeah," Baggs said. "But you'd never know it by looking at him."

After two hours of steady climbing and seven hours of rugged maneuvering on narrow rocky trails, they were ready for a good night's sleep. To Jens's surprise, this accommodation was cozy, had charcoal braziers instead of a smoky firebox, real beds, and the only potatoes they had seen since their arrival in Albania—French fries! Following the most tasty supper they had had since crash-landing, they were shown to an upstairs room and were fast asleep ten minutes after climbing between the feather ticks.

Report of Captain Lloyd G. Smith, OSS

[17 December 1943]

On the afternoon of December 17, 1943, word was received by W/T from Cairo that the party had left Progonat and were expected to be at Kuc on the 21st.

17 December 1943, Friday—0800:
En Route to Progonat

As Jens and the nurses joined the rest of the group outside, they crowded around one another as much to keep warm as to try to talk and find out who might have the latest word on anything. Neither the pilots nor Gary, Steffa, and Blondie had arrived yet.

"Has anyone talked to Gary this morning?" Jens asked.

"No," Sergeant Adams said. "I walked up to their place just now and they were busy working the set. I'm guessing they are finally getting a message from Cairo."

Steffa and two other Albanians showed up ten minutes later.

"Did all the scouts get back?" Jean asked. "What did they report? Which way are we going?"

Steffa held up his hand. He looked depressed. Usually he was very glad to have any information to hand out, but now he answered slowly. "They say there is much fighting in many directions. Gary sent scouts out again this morning, but they haven't returned. Maybe he'll decide to go on and hope we'll meet them on the trail. He and Blondie have been working the radio all night, but I don't know if they ever got through to or received a message from Cairo."

When Gary appeared at last, he looked old and tired. The black mustache he had grown since they left Krushove had added several years to his apparent age, and a sleepless night had put circles under his eyes and lines around his mouth. He nodded to the group and motioned toward the scouts. "Let's get going," he said.

Two mules appeared behind him, one with the kerosene drums tied to its sides, the other with the radio strapped to it.

They walked on without a word passing between them. Everyone was tired of speculating, and there was no news to stimulate hope or imagination.

17 December 1943, Friday—Progonat

The party stopped about noon at a small village of only four or five houses in bleak plateau country. They entered the first building they came to. It resembled a dingy saloon. After Jens's eyes accommodated to the darkness, she could see a table, some chairs in one corner of the room, and several Albanian men standing by a high bar, drinking either wine or tea. Jens moved closer so she could hear the conversation between them and Panda. Panda was having a difficult time understanding what they were saying as they all talked at once, flapping their arms excitedly, shaking their heads, and clicking their tongues.

Panda turned to the group. "There is fierce fighting going on between here and the coast."

Jens wanted to shout at him, where, exactly where? How much of the area is involved? Is it a German push toward this area?

Gary spoke to Panda. "We'll stay overnight. Tell them to make room for everyone."

They stood huddled together in that small, dimly lit building, waiting for the arrangements to be made.

Jens turned to Steffa. "Did those scouts that Gary sent out ever get back?"

He shook his head. "I haven't seen them. They probably never left to go look."

Split up five or six to a house, they had to settle down to wait again. Jens felt it was a real cat-and-mouse game, and that always being the mouse was no fun at all.

Report of Captain Lloyd G. Smith, OSS

18 December 1943
At 0900 hours on the morning of December 18, 1943, I left the Base for Kuc. I was using the coastal trail via Palasa, Dhermi, Vuno, and Piluri, since the Germans were still active around Dukati and Terbaci. . . . this was a hell of a rough trail.

Report of Lieutenant Gavin B. Duffy, SOE

[18 December 1943]
Zhulat, M. 31 to Progonat, M. 32
Messages received from Cairo at ARGYROKASTRON

[Gjirokastër] revealed a new German drive from Valona striking towards the area of Seaview, the evacuation point. However, the message from CAIRO did not, quite rightly too, order me to halt, but take all precautions.

I decided on PROGONAT as it was a day's march from the fighting area and was the only village in that huge area which had survived the blitz staged by the ITALIANS and GERMANS in turn. This day [we] did arrive and we slept at PROGONAT, the weather being bitterly cold and the way hard, much climbing, filthy tracks.

Report of Captain Lloyd G. Smith, OSS

19 December 1943

I arrived in Dhermi at 1400 hours, December 19, 1943, after spending the night in a shepherd's cave along the coast.

From Dhermi, I traveled to Vuno with the Commissar of Vuno in an automobile leaving Dhermi at 1830 hours and arriving in Vuno at 1900 hours. The Commissar reported that the Partisans were too strong to be routed out of Kuc by the Germans.

Report of Gavin B. Duffy, SOE

[19 December 1943]

The next day, I left the party at Progonat with the W/T set and set off for Kuc, the HQ for the local 'STABHIT,' arriving at Gushmare, a village two hours from PROGONAT going in the direction of KUC. I was informed that the SHADIT had moved to GOLEM which is east of KUC, so I moved back to PROGONAT, arranging for the party to stay a further night. W/T again set up sending and receiving messages.

11 By Air or by Sea?

20 December 1943, Monday—0800:
En Route to Kuc

Unexpectedly summoned to gather their belongings and leave Progonat for Kuc, the group assembled outside in anticipation of news. Jens looked in vain for Gary, Blondie, and Panda. When it was determined that everyone was present, the guides motioned for the group to follow them. Jens increased her pace to catch up to Steffa.

"Where's Gary?" she asked.

"He left with Blondie and Panda about two hours ago and will wait for us in Kuc," Steffa said.

"How far is Kuc from here?" Jens asked.

"About two and a half hours."

Jens allowed herself to fall back in the line as she pondered what Steffa had said. If Gary felt that he had to go to Kuc himself, she thought, it must mean that he doesn't trust scouts to do the job. She hoped he wasn't walking into a trap set by German sympathizers.

Before they had been on the trail a full hour they met streams of people walking in the opposite direction. They stepped aside to let the travelers pass, and Steffa talked to anyone who would stop. Most were carrying a few belongings and a child or two. Several wounded men were being transported on homemade stretchers.

Jens looked down the trail to see where the stream might end and spied Gary's familiar, quick stride among the stragglers and his black fur hat above the crowd. All of the Americans' eyes were on him as he approached. When they met, he stopped, glanced at the group, and bit his bottom lip as though he really didn't want to tell them what he had found out. It seemed to Jens that he always expected an hysterical reaction from one of the nurses and was sizing them up to figure out which one it would be. He shook his head and spoke in a clear, sober tone.

"We can't go through. They're fighting right now in Kuc, just two hours from here." He raised his voice and spoke a little louder. "We'll have to get out of this area as quickly as possible to avoid being trapped."

He struck out in the direction from which they had just come, and they turned and followed him without a word. At the pace Gary set, they overtook the stretchers, the elderly, many walking with the aid of canes, and younger people carrying children all in a matter of minutes.

The party arrived in Golem, the coldest, bleakest, most wind-swept village they had passed through. There wasn't one tree to break the cold wind that raged among the few houses in winter nor to offer shade from the scorching sun in summer. It was 1500, and Gary decided he needed to set up the wireless to inform Cairo of the fighting in and about Kuc. He left to look for a suitable house, while the group stood huddled on the outskirts of town and hoped they wouldn't have to stay the night.

While he was gone, Thrasher and Baggs brought up the possibility of air evacuation. Jens thought they must have talked it over between themselves, since their argument was organized and well presented.

"A C-47 can easily land in that grassy field we crossed," Thrasher said. "We all fit on one plane before so it shouldn't be a problem fitting on one to get out." He shrugged. "Who knows, our people may decide to send two transports for us. But if we don't ask, we'll never know."

"It sounds good to me," Jens said. "Have you mentioned it to Gary yet?"

"No. We wanted to make sure first that we all agreed on it," Baggs said. "Unless there are any objections, we'll bring it up as soon as he gets back."

Gary and Steffa returned in twenty minutes.

"I can get only one house," Gary said. "The people here don't have enough food for themselves. They're also afraid of having so many of us stay here." He paused briefly. "I'm told there's a village about two hours from here. The guides will take you there, while I stay here and contact Cairo. As soon as we get a message through, we'll join you in Kalonja."

Thrasher interrupted him, announced their plan, and asked for his opinion. Gary looked at the pilots as if they had taken leave of their senses.

"We can't do that," he said.

"Why not?" Thrasher asked. "That grassy field we crossed near Gjirokastër—Steffa said the Italians used it as an airfield, and it's plenty big enough for a C-47. We'll make up a message for you to send out tonight, if you want."

"No, I don't want, and if you send any such message, you will direct it to your own air force headquarters, or whoever may be in command," Gary said.

"Well, okay," Baggs said. "We can address it to 'Commander of the Twelfth Air Force.'"

"Do you realize who that is?" Gary asked. Before Baggs could answer, Thrasher spoke up. "General Spaatz," he said. "That's okay. I don't mind asking him for a lift on one of his C-47s under these circumstances."

"I have my orders," Gary said, "and they are to get you people to the coast safely."

"We'll take responsibility for this," Thrasher said.

"You're damn right you will," Gary snapped. He looked at the rest of the group. "You'd better get going. As it is, you'll be walking part way in the dark." He nodded toward two Albanian men. "These guides know where to take you. I'll join you as soon as possible."

The Americans took off down the trail and Jens didn't realize for thirty minutes that the pilots, Steffa, and Panda were not with them.

It was pitch-dark before they reached Kalonja, and a cold drizzle had begun to fall. A woman answered their knock on the door of the first house they came to, and a young teenage boy, probably her son, joined her. The guides spoke to them for about fifteen minutes while the group got colder and soaked to the skin. Finally, they were admitted to the house and crowded into one room. They had not eaten all day, and had had only a swallow or two of water from their canteens. No food or water was offered to them. They pulled off their wet shoes and socks and sat on the floor around the fire, trying to get warm.

"My feet are just about healed. Thank God for the British Mission," Tooie said.

The sergeants informed the group that guards had been posted around the village and would fire a single rifle shot if an enemy were approaching.

"It's a wonder that Owen and Allen could arrange for the guards since we don't have anyone with us who speaks Albanian," Jens said. "I can't believe Gary sent us off without an interpreter."

"Thank goodness, we'll be asleep for the night and won't need a translator," Jean said.

"Let's hope we don't," Jens answered.

Report of Lieutenant Gavin B. Duffy, SOE

[20 December 1943]

The following day I informed Lieutenant Thrasher that I was again going ahead and he was to bring the party two hours after. I arrived at Gushmare—what chaos I witnessed here! The partisan hospital was being evacuated. Myself being a victim of many desert flaps! From 1941 to 1942, this appeared like our own guns flying through my unit leagur.

This was enough, I waited for party to arrive which [with] wounded partisans of the first brigade who just had not been quick enough. I gathered them together as calmly as possible, and told them we would have to go back. They were at this point only two days from their goal—so heartbreaking surely! . . . So we ended after a great and tiresome struggle our first attempt at evacuation. As events proved later, the German drive was an avalanche.

Report of Captain Lloyd G. Smith, OSS

20 December 1943
  Picking up two Partisan guides at Vuno, I left for Pilurit 0700 hours on December 20, 1943 and arrived there at 1130 hours—I left Piluri for Kuc at 1200 hours and noticed many Italian soldiers on their way back from Kuc. I was stopped by Partisans about one mile from Kuc at 1430 hours and told that Germans had occupied Kuc that morning. The Germans had come up from Borshi and down from Terbaci. I left immediately for Piliuri and arrived there at 1700 hours. Weather bad with heavy rain.

21 December 1943, Tuesday—0145: Kalonja

The crack of a single rifle shot ripped the group from sleep. Jens lay in her spot on the floor a moment too long. Several of the sergeants in the back of the room ran forward toward the door, treating Jens as part of the floor.

"Wait a minute!" Jens shouted. "You're walking on me!" She scrambled to her feet and followed her companions outside, listening for further sounds. Three of the sergeants disappeared into the darkness.

After fifteen minutes, they returned from checking with the guards.

"False alarm!" Sergeant Allen announced. "Somebody got a little trigger-happy. Go back to sleep."

They made their way back into the room and reclaimed their places on the cold floor. Despite the excitement, they were sound asleep again within twenty minutes—with their boots on.

The second rifle shot roused them two hours later. This time Jens was one of the first people out the door. Allen, Adams, and Owen hurried into the dark night to check on the guards and returned within twenty minutes. "Another false alarm," Sergeant Allen said. "Keep your boots on, and try to go back to sleep."

"If that guy fires his rifle one more time in a false alarm, I'm going to borrow a gun and shoot him myself," Jens said.

"You'll have to get in line for that honor," Jean called from across the room.

It was daylight when Jens awakened. Several nurses and sergeants were already sitting up and carrying on a conversation in hushed tones.

The woman who had greeted them at the door the previous night walked into the room, spoke in Albanian, and motioned toward the outside door.

"Does anyone know what she's saying?" Lois asked.

"I don't understand a word, but I'm pretty sure she wants us to leave," Sergeant Allen said. "They didn't want us here in the first place."

"We can't leave," Jens said. "We have to wait here for Gary. We sure don't need to take off on our own."

"Germani! Germani!" the woman said excitedly. She pulled an index finger across her throat then pointed to the door again. "Germani!"

They sat and looked at the woman as if they did not comprehend the message behind her words and gestures.

"I certainly understand how she feels, and why she'd like us to leave," Tooie said.

"We all do," Jens said. "But we can't leave without Gary. She'll just have to put up with us for a while."

Sergeant Allen stood up and made a sweeping motion with his right arm, as though ushering someone into the room. "Po. Po," he said. "Germani! Po. Po!"

The woman looked shocked, and stared at Allen as if he were crazy. He repeated his gesture and words.

"I think she's getting the idea, Allen," Jens said. "We're not leaving until we see the whites of the enemies' eyes."

The woman threw up her arms, said a few words in a disgusted tone, and walked out of the room.

"I hope Gary gets here before they decide to throw us out physically," Tooie said.

At 1335 Steffa and the pilots walked in the door. Before they could say more than hello, several people told them what they thought about being sent ahead without an interpreter. An understanding was reached that with two interpreters, one would go with the group if Gary had to send the Americans ahead again. Of course the understanding depended on Gary's approval.

"Did Gary send the message about an air evacuation?" Jens asked.

"Yeah," Baggs said. "He finally agreed to let us sign our names, but he would have nothing to do with the request." He sat down near the fire. "I imagine the British will have the first right of refusal. I guess with the weather like this, it won't matter anyway."

Gary arrived at Kalonja just before dark and arranged for the party to spend a second night, despite the protestations of the owner of the house.

Report of Captain Lloyd G. Smith, OSS

21 December 1943
   On the next morning, (December 21, 1943) I left Piluri for Vuno at 0645 hours. It was still raining on arrival at Vuno at 1330 hours. Before entering Vuno, I studied the town and the highway through the field glasses from the top of a hill. During fifteen minutes of observation, I saw two heavy MTs pulling guns through the town. After making sure that there were no Germans posted in the town, I went on in to the Partisan headquarters. During my stay in Vuno, a total of six heavy trucks drawing 75 mm guns and one command car full of Germans passed through, going north. My observations were made from a house alongside the road.
   At 1930 hours, I left Vuno for Dhermi, arriving at 2000 hours. I slept at Dhermi that night.

22 December 1943, Wednesday—0815: En Route to Doksat

The party arose early and Gary hustled them on their way. The rain had turned to sleet, and before the day was half over their clothing had been soaked through. Their socks were saturated with cold water.

At sunset they stopped at a village called Karla and were surprised to find crowds of people milling about in the cold night air. As they walked into the town, Jens heard a familiar voice.

"Meester Baggs, Meester Baggs!"

She turned and saw Hassan running toward the party. His familiar black cape flapped about his knees as he ran; his rifle bounced up and down on his back.

"Meester Baggs!" he yelled again as he raced to the copilot and grabbed him in a big bear hug. He laughed, talked and patted him on the back, then stepped away and tweaked Baggs's reddish mustache. "Very beautiful!" he said and laughed again.

"Hassan, Hassan!" others in their party cried and came to greet him. He seemed genuinely pleased with their excitement at seeing him and tried to grasp each hand.

"Is this part of your area?" Jens asked.

"No, but maybe I make it mine," he grinned his knowing smile. "Germans take all my territory last week. So we move farther south." He shrugged and added, "Maybe later we go back again."

As they talked, he was looking around the group for someone. Finally he asked, "Where is Ann?" He knew only her first name but gestured to indicate her five-foot-nine-inch height and the long hair that she wore wrapped around her head.

"I don't know," Jens answered. "We haven't seen her since we left Berat the morning the Germans came into the town."

"You were still there when Germans came?"

"Yes. We left quickly that morning. Everything was pretty confused," Jens said. "When we got together later, Ann Maness and two other girls were missing. As far as we could figure out, they never left Berat."

"Oh," he said in a low voice. "Too bad to Ann. I like her very much!" He shook his head. "Germans are very bad. Maybe I soon teach them a lesson for Ann."

"How's that?" Jens asked.

"Maybe one of the open cars carrying their officers get blown up. It happened before to them, maybe it will happen again very soon."

"Isn't that awfully dangerous for you? What if you get caught?" Jens asked.

"I throw stick of dynamite and disappear like the wind," Hassan said. "I not get caught." He grinned.

Before Jens could comment further, Gary called the party together, and they were led in groups of four and five to individual houses for the night.

Report of Captain Lloyd G. Smith, OSS

22 December 1943

The next morning (December 22, 1943), it was still raining and since my clothes were still wet, I decided to stay in Dhermi that day. At about 1700 hours, I received word that the Germans were making a house to house search of Vuno for Partisans and weapons. Suspecting that Dhermi would be next on their list, I moved to a house at the extreme western end of town and made ready for a fast get-a-way. In the meantime, it was still raining. At 2200 hours, I received word that 80 Germans had arrived Dhermi and had started a house to house search for Partisans. I accordingly moved from Dhermi to a cave southwest of Palasa and spent the remainder of the night sleeping there with a shepherd and his flock.

23 December 1943, Thursday—0810: En Route to Doksat

In the morning Jens, Tooie, and Jean looked for Hassan and his crowd and learned that they had left Karla at 0700. By 0830 Jens and the rest were headed again for Doksat.

When they reached the river that they had crossed on their way to Kuc, the boatman were huddled together against the cold. They seemed glad to pull the Americans across the water in the same flat, shallow boat that had carried them the other way some days earlier. The bridge was still intact and the road was quiet as they ran along it and down a bank to flat land that led to the grassy airfield. This time, Thrasher and Baggs spent some time looking it over and walking it off to see if it was smooth enough for a C-47 to land and if there were any signs that it might be mined.

They arrived at Doksat in the late afternoon. It seemed a pleasant little town, with stone streets and narrow, shelflike sidewalks. The party was divided again into threes, fours, and fives and led to individual houses. Elna, Marky, and Jens were taken to a house where three people were standing in the doorway. Jens wondered if they were there to welcome them or ask them to move on to another village. She was relieved when the young woman, breaking into a smile, extended her hand and beckoned them to come inside. The older couple followed; they seemed to do so reluctantly, but as though not to be outdone in hospitality, they motioned to a bench in front of a roaring fire. The nurses took off their trenchcoats, removed their wet shoes and socks, and dried their feet in front of the fireplace. This done, Jens turned her attention to the house.

The living room was long, with windows facing the street and a door that opened right onto the sidewalk. The room was spacious, and Jens tried to figure out what, besides its dimensions, was so different about it. Then it occurred to her. The fire was blazing without adding smoke to the room. Jens was further delighted when the old couple returned, smiling, and handed each nurse an orange. The fresh fruit was a special treat to the weary trekkers, who ate them slowly, savoring every morsel.

Gary had sent a message to Cairo, but had not received an answer in Golem. No matter, Jens thought, the weather was foul with rain and sleet, and thick clouds were hanging low over the mountaintops.

Report of Captain Lloyd G. Smith, OSS

23 December 1943

On the following morning (December 23, 1943) at 0500 hours with rain still falling, I left the cave for the Base where I arrived at 1700 hours.

In the meantime, Cdr. Glen had received a message that the American Party had retraced their steps from Kuc to Golem because of the German activity in that section.

Report of Lieutenant Gavin B. Duffy, SOE

23 December 1943

Myself with party and W/T set now at DOKSAT, waiting from CAIRO, the answer to a message sent re pick-up planes. The pilots had inspected the airfield and pronounced it as suitable, and their report had been passed to CAIRO. By this time, the weather was filthy, the complete valley was enshrouded in thick soup, ground visibility was not more than 100 yards.

A brief sitrep was sent to CAIRO each day examples: DDD. No. 13 of 23

"From Duffy party due at Doksat rpt DOKSAT tomorrow. Am sending two pilots to inspect field. Self will confer with TILMAN to make final arrangements for pickup. As weather bad have made clear to YANKS they take full responsibility for aircraft. Ends" DDD.

"From DUFFY weather still bad waiting for break before stating time of pickup. All party ready what news TILMAN still waiting."

The only thing which was holding off the pickup at this time was the weather. The main highway running past ARGYROKASTRON and the airfield was clear. My office was quite clear as to the position here and knew that planes were not to be sent unless my O.K. was received.

24 December 1943, Friday—1930: Doksat

They threaded their way along the pitch-dark, cobblestone street, whispering so they could keep track of one another. If the moon were anywhere, it couldn't shine through the heavy, low cloud cover. Steffa led the group to the house where the pilots were staying. They had decided that they should all get together for Christmas Eve.

Jens was a little reluctant to have everyone under one roof again because there had been so much squabbling among them over the past week. Their disagreements had been exacerbated by the many setbacks, foul weather, and illness. One big tiff had developed over several cartons of cigarettes that two of the women had hoarded. The British had given them the cartons to take along when they left Krushove. Jens's guess was that the British had meant them to be shared, but these two had decided that the cigarettes had been given to them and had placed the cartons in a suitcase. Gary had insisted that some of the men should carry it, so they had helplessly handed it over, even though before Gary had joined them, they had settled on a rule that each person would carry his or her own belongings.

They had even quarreled about food they didn't have. A menu of steak, mashed potatoes, a big green salad, buttered peas, rolls with butter, and strawberry shortcake with mounds of whipped cream, served with piping hot coffee, was voted their favorite meal. They talked about it as the first meal they would have once they had been evacuated; they dreamed about it in Technicolor. Then one day Elna mentioned that she would love to have a big bowl of steaming hot oatmeal topped with lots of sugar, real cream, and cold, sliced peaches. The group attacked her as if she had said she'd like to remain in Albania and thought everyone should do the same.

"How could anyone prefer oatmeal to steak?" Jean asked.

Everyone agreed that anyone with taste would choose steak and vowed again to make it their first meal after leaving Albania.

It sure won't be our Christmas dinner, Jens thought. In fact, we'll all count ourselves lucky to have any food at all on Christmas Day.

The group stopped in front of the house where the pilots were staying. It looked totally dark until they opened the front door. As the group entered a dimly lit room, Jens's eyes went immediately to a small cedar bough perched on a tiny table in the corner of the room, decked out in small red ribbon bows.

"Wherever did you get decorations?" Jens asked.

Tooie smiled, "We found the bough, and one of us just happened to have a piece of ribbon in her musette bag."

The "tree" added a festive note and gave the group new and positive excitement that it badly needed.

Lois came in, sat down, and fluffed her hair. "I got the nicest

Christmas present," she said. "My hair washed, the second time since November the eighth."

"Elna, Marky, and I are whistling clean too," Jens said. "But these filthy clothes will have to go to church tomorrow!"

"Who's going to church tomorrow?" Lois asked.

"You mean you aren't, you lucky dog. Maybe you're living with non-churchgoers," Jens said.

"But I'd like to go," she insisted.

"At 5:00 A.M.?"

"Oh," she gasped. "In that case tell me all about it sometime."

"Who are you going with, and to what church?" Jean asked.

Steffa answered the question. "The Greek Orthodox is the only church here."

"The only church in the country?" Elna asked.

"There are a few Catholic churches yet, but as you know by now, at least 70 percent of the people are of the Muslim faith," Steffa replied.

Jens pointed at Steffa. "He got us into this."

Steffa smiled. "You didn't have to say yes. I only repeated what the lady of the house asked you."

"My curiosity got the best of me—until I learned the service is at 5:00 A.M." Jens looked at Steffa. "Besides, I felt the family was doing something special by asking us, so I thought we really ought to go."

"Yes," Steffa said. "They were very pleased that you want to go with them."

"Well, with any luck, my curiosity will last until the service is over."

As they sat around the fire, most of the party told stories of previous Christmases. For many of the young sergeants, this was their first Christmas away from home. They wondered aloud about their younger brothers and sisters and told of the last time they had watched as the kids tore into their presents.

Suddenly Sergeant Adams shouted, "Let's sing Christmas carols!"

"Yes," Steffa said, "please sing 'Hark the Herald Angels Sing,' first. I haven't heard carols sung by a group that really knows them for many years now."

"You're taking a lot for granted if you think we know all of them," Lois said.

They sang all the carols they could think of, and Steffa invariably knew more verses than they did. "Mr. Fultz taught them to us in the Albanian-American School and I never forgot them. I have taught them to my wife and children too."

About 2300 the nurses got up to leave. Gary got to his feet, smiled, and said, "We must sing 'God Save the King,' you know."

"Only if we sing the 'Star-Spangled Banner' too," Elna said.

Gary looked around and said, "Well, I'm a bit outnumbered tonight."

The Yanks sang the "Star-Spangled Banner" and hummed along to "God Save the King." Everyone was in a gay mood and started singing again as they went out the door. The more cautious admonished, "We aren't in the States, and I don't think it pays to advertise our presence here."

When they reached their assigned house, Elna, Marky, and Jens slipped quietly upstairs and between feather ticks on the floor. The next thing Jens knew, the young daughter-in-law of the house was shaking them awake. They climbed into their slacks without getting out from beneath the feather ticks.

The night air was frigid and damp. Steffa met them as they approached the small church with the family. They stayed at the back while the family went forward to the pews, which were little boxes without kneelers, each large enough for three or four people.

Steffa tried to explain some of the service to them. Jens could get only a glimpse of the priests and some of his assistants, as they went through the ritual. Part of the sermon had once been delivered in Latin, but since their break with Rome it was now in Greek and Albanian, according to Steffa. The sky showed faint streaks of light as they walked "home" and went right back to bed.

25 December 1943, Saturday—1915: Doksat

On Christmas night Gary and Blondie sent word for everyone to join them at their assigned house. They had a couple of bottles of wine and rochi. They drank a toast to Christmas, the New Year, and "the coast." Again, they talked about Christmases with their families before they entered the military. Gary listened to the stories of younger sisters and brothers with rapt attention. He laughed and shook his head. "You know, I've never been around women very much. I don't even have sisters."

"You're getting them in large doses now," Jens said. "Do you think we're here to stay?"

He laughed again. "I must admit that when I was first given the assignment to evacuate a group that included ten nurses, I almost turned tail and ran. However, when I met you and learned that you had already been through quite a bit since you crash-landed and were still in good spirits, I felt sure—God willing—that I could get you to the coast." He looked around the group and added, "You know, you girls really have a lot of guts."

"Thank you," Marky said. She smiled at him. "Where in England do you live?"

"Leeds. That's in the north, but actually I'm from Dublin. My family has a home there too."

Steffa, ever aware of world history, piped up, "But Mister Gary, if you're Irish, what are you doing in a British uniform?"

Gary's eyes narrowed and his lips tightened. "Now let's get this war over before we start that one all over again!"

Everyone laughed good-naturedly at Gary. He was not only intense—he was truly unique!

No one asked if there had been any recent messages on the wireless or if the fighting were still going on. The last word they had received on Captain Lloyd Smith was that he had left the area and gone back to the coast. Gary was relaxed and talkative again, and everyone was reluctant to break the Christmas mood, preferring that reality not come crashing in on this one night.

They did speak of Lytle, Maness, and Porter, and, as always, wondered where they were and what they were doing.

"Don't you think it's strange that we haven't heard about them at all?" Jens asked. "Do you think they were captured?"

"No," Gary said. "I doubt it. *That* I believe we would have heard about. They're most likely holed up, and it's just as well if we don't ask a lot of questions about them. If the Germans don't hear about them, they'll assume you're all still together and not search for them."

"I guess you're right, but how will they make contact with anyone?" Marky asked.

"Just as you did. They'll have to send word with somebody, and maybe they feel it isn't safe to do that yet."

Report of Captain Lloyd G. Smith, OSS

26 December 1943

At this time, I also received a message from Bari dated December 26, 1943, instructing me to come out on the next boat.

27 December 1943, Monday—0845: Doksat

Jens was one of the last to awaken the next day and went right to the window to check on the weather. The clouds had lifted considerably, raising her hopes for a clear sky. Elna and Marky were sitting by the fire when she went downstairs.

"So, what's new?" she asked as she sat down beside them.

"We've been trying to figure that out," Marky said.

"Why?"

"People have been appearing alone and in groups of three or four for the last hour or two," Elna said.

"Maybe it's just visiting day," Jens suggested.

"Hardly. No one has set foot in here yet," Marky said.

A knock on the front door interrupted their conversation, and the man of the house burst through from the kitchen area as if he had been waiting for it. A younger man entered, and the two went directly to the kitchen.

By noon the village was bustling with people arriving every few minutes, but most of them remained outside. Often as not, they spoke to the host of the house through a half-open door.

There was another knock, and Jens could see Gary's fur cap through the opening. He and Blondie and Panda walked in quickly.

"Are we glad to see you!" Elna said. "Or are you just following the customs too?"

"What customs?" Gary asked.

"We decided that they must go calling here on the days just after Christmas, because they've had a stack of visitors already," Marky said.

"Did they try to tell you, or have you heard at all what's going on?"

"Going on?" Elna said. "Where?"

"The Germans took over Gjirokastër this morning!" Gary said.

"What?" The nurses stood there with their mouths open.

"Is there a window up there?" Gary pointed to the stairs. "Can you see Gjirokastër from it?"

"Are you kidding?" Jens said. "All we've seen out that window is clouds." She followed Gary up the stairs.

He stood in front of the only window in the bedroom and held his field glasses to his eyes.

Jens could see much farther now. "Is that Gjirokastër perched on that hill? It must be," she answered herself.

"Quite a few vehicles going in, mostly trucks," Gary said to Blondie, who was standing next to him. "A few cars and now and again a half-track." He gave the glasses to Blondie.

After a long silence, Blondie said, "I don't see anything that looks like heavy weapons, but who can tell what's in those trucks!"

"How could they drive into that town? The streets are nothing but wide steps," Jens said.

"Oh, there's a road into town—just one I'm sure," Gary said. "So all they haul in has to come out the same way." He took the glasses from Blondie and watched.

Jens turned to Panda. "What have you heard? Why did they decide to take the town? Has the fighting come this way?"

He thought a moment and answered in his slow, ponderous way. "People who came here from Gjirokastër earlier today said that dynamite was thrown into a car full of German officers yesterday, and this is retaliation for it."

"What a shame that the whole town is punished for one action," Jens said.

"That's their favorite target, a car full of German officers," Gary said without taking the field glasses from his eyes or moving his head.

"We must fight them wherever we have a chance," Panda said with emphasis.

Jens, thinking of the misery brought to an entire town by the rash deed of some hotheads, suddenly remembered Hassan's pantomime of a car full of German officers. His words echoed in her mind: "All smoking cigars until we throw a stick of dynamite, and then Germani smoke all over!" He had laughed as if he were speaking of a practical joke.

After Gary, Blondie, and Panda had gone, Thrasher and Baggs came in with their field glasses. The nurses showed them the upstairs window, and they all watched Gjirokastër. There was a steady stream of vehicles. Baggs sat on the window seat and wiped his eyes. "If this weather would just clear before they get too much heavy stuff in there and set up! We don't even know how much heavy stuff they have in the country, and if the British know, Gary isn't telling. It's for sure they can't have it in any of those vehicles unless it's dismantled, and if that's so, they'll need time to put it together again." He bit his lower lip. "This could raise hell with our air evac plans. If the Krauts get anything much set up there, they'll be in a perfect position, looking right down on the field where the planes are supposed to land."

"Damn!" Elna said. "It's just like Berat. How can they get into our hair so unwittingly? Just when we need one of those towns for a few days, boom, it all blows up!"

"I hope it is unwittingly," Marky said. "You don't suppose they know about our plans to bring planes in, do you? I mean, I suppose they could eventually break our code and intercept our messages."

"Don't even think that!" Elna said.

"That isn't likely," Baggs said. "It's probably just a retaliation for the officers who were blown up."

They left, saying they'd be back later. "We'll see if we can help Gary with his wireless. He's having a lot of trouble with it because of the weather."

"Not again!" Elna said. "Radio trouble and bad weather is where this all got started."

28 December 1943, Tuesday—0900: Doksat

For the next two days they could see only a hundred yards away in the fog and could only guess at what was going on. Visitors arrived in a steady stream, and rumors were rampant. Three of the sergeants came with glasses to look out the window. They tried to sound encouraging and said they didn't think the Germans had heavy equipment in the country.

"Yeah, but they do have antiaircraft guns. Remember the road to Berat?" Jens asked.

Gary came in, bounded up the stairs to convince himself that he couldn't see the town, and came right back down. "Damn, I'd like to know what's going on." He sat down on the bench with Marky, Elna, and Jens.

"What are the refugees saying?" Jens asked.

"They all say the same thing. The Germans are there, taking over everything, but nothing about what I'm interested in. They only wanted to get out! I even sent people who should be able to walk around the town and talk to anyone without too much trouble," he said.

"What do they report back?" Elna asked.

"Oh, just what all the refugees say, that the Germans are moving in, but not with how much or what kind of stuff." He gave one of his disgusted grunts. "They never go into town, you can be very sure of that—they're too cowardly. They're doing exactly what Panda and Steffa are doing for me here, talking to the refugees. They just stay away several hours and then repeat their stories."

"One of the sergeants told us that there is a rumor that Smith has been captured," Elna said.

"That would be difficult for me to believe," Gary said. "Smith is trained to take care of himself. Don't believe everything you hear. Rumors are less reliable than this country's weather."

Report of Lieutenant Gavin B. Duffy, SOE

28 December 1943
Everything looked nice and rosy until the 27th of Decem-

ber. Small party of Germans from DELVINE entered
ARGYROKASTRON [Gjirokastër], looting several of the
shops and preparing to leave. They did on the afternoon of
the 27th, send a truck and motor cycle away back from the
town, plus the loot to DELVINE, this complement was
unfortunately attacked by partisans who did allow some of
them to escape.

I opened up with CAIRO on the 20.00 hrs sked and failed
to make contact, as on several occasions my operator Sgt.
BELL used to get CAIRO "blaring" in at fives! But himself
was not heard.

28 December 1943, Tuesday—1810: Doksat

There was very little conversation as Marky, Elna, and Jens sat and
ate the soup that was brought to them in a large tin pan. A few long
bones, dark gray and greasy, floated in the liquid. They decided the
bones were from a goat, and that it was these bones that gave the
soup its pungent odor and flavor.

There was a quick knock. The family didn't respond, so Jens
started for the door. Before she got there, it was opened slowly, and
Thrasher and Baggs came in and joined them by the fire.

"Gary got a message from Cairo," Baggs said quietly. "It was
pretty garbled, as usual, but a C-47 or maybe two, with fighters, will
arrive at 1300 tomorrow."

"Do you mean it? You wouldn't kid us, now would you? And
what about the weather?" They pelted him with one question after
another.

"Do they know about the Germans?"

"Gary has been reporting about them in every message, but the
Heinies have been so successful with jamming all the messages coming this way that we have no confirmation on it. This message barely
came through," Thrasher said. "Gary's trying now to get and give
more information—it may take all night."

In spite of this long-awaited good news, they weren't jubilant;
there were still too many "ifs" and Gary, they knew, had been dead

set against the air evacuation plan even without the Germans. Baggs and Thrasher both seemed tense and fidgety.

"What about the weather? The clouds were right on the mountain tops this afternoon."

"I know," Thrasher said quietly, "but they must be getting a clear weather report for this area for tomorrow, or they wouldn't be setting up this flight."

They edged toward the door. "We'd better go tell the rest of the gang," Baggs said. "Unless you hear differently, let's be ready to start by 0900. It's a good two-hour walk, but that should give us plenty of time to reach the field."

"Don't worry," Jens said. "We'll be there with bells on!"

Report of Lieutenant Gavin B. Duffy, SOE

[28 December 1943]

By this time things were getting desperate. The weather had taken a sudden change and was perfect. On the 28th, failed to make contact with CAIRO, until on the 20.00 hrs sked; they had some messages for us; transmission was bad. Sgt. BELL could just hear CAIRO and they were changing him to every frequency; *NOTE:* On one occasion, he was asked to change to a frequency he had ceased to use, five months previously.

The Messages.

I took his first one and deciphered it as follows:

"The following arrangements will hold for PU of YANKS. PU between 11.00 GMT and 13.00 GMT Wed Dec 28th [29th]. If weather prevents will try again sometime next two successive days have party completely ready At. SE. corner of field.

"Permit no person within mile of Airfield except your party and one strong partisan guard group to stay with your party. Confirm O.K. QRZ. at 21.30 GMT tonight."

Contact was tried again later in the evening with our QRX 23.45 but failed. Lt. THRASHER can confirm how CAIRO used to come blaring in. It was impossible to confirm QRX 21.30, as it was not received due heavy atmospherics until close on QRX request and still had to be deciphered.

Again chaos reigned in the village. The locals, after the partisans' attack, were expecting reprisals. I tried to get a man to leave DOKSAT for bringing information from inside ARGYROKASTRON. At 02.00 hrs, I succeeded in getting one of the locals to go for the payment of one sov.

29 December 1943, Wednesday—0815: Doksat to Gjirokastër

They awakened early the next morning and scrambled for the window to look at the sky. It was almost clear; the clouds were high overhead, and they could see Gjirokastër again. There was a little ground haze, but that would burn off with the sun, they were sure.

Their hosts were more than a little relieved that they were leaving, no matter how suddenly. They had been there nearly a week, and with the events of the past few days, the locals didn't need stranded Americans to complicate their lives further. Jens felt quite sure they couldn't know anything about the planes, as word had come quite late the previous day. As they thanked their hosts, the young woman hugged the three nurses goodbye.

The party gathered in the small town square and waited for Gary. "Can you believe they're really coming for us?" Sergeant Allen said. "Can you believe it?"

"I'm more surprised that Gary is allowing them to come," Sergeant Cruise said.

Marky, who was standing nearby, put her finger to her lips and whispered, "Shh, let's just pray all goes well for everyone's sake!"

Gary looked tired and tense as he approached. He glanced around at everyone with scarcely a nod, then stopped at a distance and spoke to Blondie. Jens studied his face and the faces of the pilots. Whether by design or not, their expressions said nothing about what they expected. Gary turned to address the group.

"Thrasher will show you the way to the field. I will meet you there shortly after you arrive." Then he turned and, in the company of Panda, struck out at his usual quick but deliberate pace.

Although they had allowed plenty of time to reach the field, they raced along and were on a high ridge overlooking the whole area by 1130, when Thrasher called for a rest stop. It was still a good half-hour's walk to the edge of the field. From their vantage point they could see a wide valley far below, beyond the bridge they'd crossed twice, and where they had followed the river as it bent around the mountain.

"Isn't it amazing how clear it is today after ten days of absolutely foul weather?" Sergeant Adams said. He scanned the sky. "I wonder which direction they'll come from."

"How long will it take to fly to Italy from here?" Elna asked.

"Probably less than an hour," Sergeant Allen said. "When we land, I intend to kiss the ground in celebration."

"That makes two of us," Sergeant Cruise said.

After a few minutes Gary and Panda arrived to join the group. Gary motioned four of the sergeants over to talk with him. Jens wondered if they were the ones who would signal the planes to land. Baggs had told them that the plan was for three or four of the men to lie on one end of the field and wait until they heard the planes. If Gary signaled them, they would stand and hold up strips of yellow parachute silk.

Then Gary moved aside to talk to Steffa and the two pilots. Jens tried to read Steffa's face to see if he had gotten the final "yes," but he walked off without betraying any emotion. When Gary began to talk with Panda, Jens felt sure he must be planning to leave. They'll say goodbye now, Jens thought, but they didn't shake hands, or make any gesture she could even guess at. Everyone else in the group was watching them too. They looked at one another for an answer or hopeful word, but nobody spoke.

Thrasher and Baggs left Gary and joined the group. They didn't look happy. Thrasher spoke in somber tones. "Gary has decided not to signal the planes to land." He looked from face to face. "He feels it's too risky with the Germans occupying Gjirokastër. He's afraid the planes would get shot up, and we'd lose some of our people too." He drew in a deep breath and stood gazing into the distance. "We won't go down any closer to the field," he said with an air of finality.

"But," Tooie said almost in tears, "if they know the town is occupied, they'll take extra precautions, won't they?"

Baggs shook his head, "I don't know, Tooie. I guess he's afraid that they really *don't* know. If the messages they got from us weren't any clearer than those we received, Gary's probably right." He sounded completely resigned.

Jens felt a heavy sickening lump in the pit of her stomach and sat down on the ground. In a strange way, she was almost relieved. At least Gary's decision had ended the guessing.

They sat numbed and looking at each other. There was nothing more to say. Jens stretched out on her back and watched the clouds racing by above her.

"Listen! Listen!" Sergeant Allen jumped to his feet. "They're coming! They're coming!" he shouted and waved his arms as he kept repeating his words.

Sergeant Zeiber tapped him on the shoulder. "We aren't going with them, you know. So don't burst a blood vessel."

"I know, but I can't wait to see some good ol' American planes anyway."

The roar of the engines filled the air and got louder by the second. All eyes were turned in the direction of the sound. The Americans scrambled to their feet and saw the whole valley suddenly fill with planes.

"Look at those fighters! Man, there are hundreds of them, hundreds!" Allen kept repeating his words. "P-38s, no less!"

"C-47s!" Cruise shouted. "Two C-47s!"

The P-38s flew back and forth over the transports. Jens tried to count them. Six, nine, twelve—she couldn't keep them separate.

Suddenly three P-38s swept low across the grassy field. As they pulled up, one flew straight on, and the other two fanned out in opposite directions—one over Gjirokastër and the other right over their heads. Three more followed in a beautifully precise formation as the first three fell in at the rear for another pass. The two C-47s had their wheels down and were headed right in for a landing as the pilots searched for those yellow strips of parachute silk to tell them the group was there and it was safe to touch down. Then, like the P-38s, they pulled up and circled.

"Hey, look!" Sergeant Owen called out. "Look at that big plane circling over Gjirokastër!"

"It's a bomber," Sergeant Adams shouted. "A four-engine job!"

Jens couldn't take her eyes off the P-38s. They continued following through in their pattern of threes, sweeping the area, then pulling up and circling back. They were beautiful, graceful planes—the fighters the Germans had come to dread. Jens could see every detail and felt sure that if the pilots looked down, they could see the group.

The C-47s came around again, wheels down, almost touching the grass before they pulled up for their final pass. If we were only at the edge of the field! Jens thought. The Germans haven't fired a shot! I'll bet we could have jumped aboard, but it's too late now.

They left just as they had come, flying low through the valley. Jens stood and watched them until they were only specks in the sky. Tears ran down her cheeks. They'll be in Italy in an hour, she thought. She wondered if any of their squadron mates would be out to greet the planes' return, or if they even knew of their mission. It was hard to believe that the Army Air Forces would put out so much equipment for only twenty-seven people. Humbling in a way, she thought. Jens could hear someone sobbing near by.

Sergeant Allen threw his cap on the ground and shook his fist at Gjirokastër, shouting, "The cowards, they didn't even fire a shot! Well, by damn, if the army thinks that much of us, we've just got to make it back!"

"I counted them," Sergeant Adams said. "There were eighteen P-38s, two C-47s, and one Wellington bomber." He grinned. "I'd say our army really does want us back."

Poor Gary, Jens thought. He won't know what to do with a bunch of tear-stained females. Baggs walked over and looked at Tooie. "If I'd even guessed they would send all that . . . but by then it was too late. We were too far from the field."

They stood around, looking at Gjirokastër and the valley until Gary called the group together. He appeared even closer to tears than many of the Americans. "Let's go back to the village," he said.

"We couldn't warn them before we left, so I hope they'll take us in again." He walked on ahead.

Jens's feet felt like lead and the journey back to the village seemed endless. When she looked at her watch, it was 1430. The planes would just be touching down in Italy.

The people gasped as they saw the Americans at their doors again, but after Steffa talked to them for a few minutes, they became quite sympathetic. Marky, Elna, and Jens returned to the house where they had stayed and sat on the bench in front of the fire. It hardly seemed as if they'd left. By bedtime the whole village knew of the attempted air rescue.

Report of Lieutenant Gavin B. Duffy, SOE

[29 December 1943]

The 0800 hours sked on the 29th failed again, so I had no option but to try the pick-up. I moved off myself to the airfield, looking at ARGYROKASTRON through binoculars. I saw the place alive with GERMANS, tanks, armd. cars, trucks and troops. They had occupied the Castle. The party arrived later at a prearranged rendezvous.

I informed them the pickup as far as they were concerned, was off and allowed them to view the GERMANS. The runner I had sent to ARGYROKASTRON arrived, full of details. Just at this time, three trucks and one armd car came down from inside the town and settled themselves on the main road near the air field. The time now was just after 12.00 hrs, so we just sat to wait in case the planes came, they did, my God! We first sighted them after hearing the noise for quite a while, coming from the direction of TEPELENE.

A perfect air display. Groups of three P.38 Lockheed nose to tail, supplying flank cover for the one Wellington and two transports, they also had ceiling cover, supplied by further groups of P.38. The "Wimpie" led the way down the huge valley about fifty feet from the ground. One or two of the nurses did break down after seeing this too perfect air display. Just imagine the feeling, seeing the transports make three

"passes" at the field, so near and yet so far—it almost seemed
that you could touch the planes, they were so low. The nurses
had unquestionably suffered a very hard time—this was
indeed too much. The planes flew around for over 15 mins,
but I would not bring them in; never in my whole life have I
been faced with such a decision. If I had brought them in,
here was the picture: three heavy planes on the air field and
the GERMANS not 500 yards away with tanks and guns! Did
the Germans fire! At the planes, no! Would they have fired at
stationary planes, who knows? I was certainly not going to
have three planes jeopardized. Maybe the first plane might
have made it, who knows! But I am sure that the other two
would not, and my job was to escort and deliver twenty-seven
bodies, not a third of the party. I was in charge of the party
and entirely responsible. You can be well assured as recent
events have shown. One has a full time job looking after
oneself in ALBANIA without having attachments, female or
otherwise. I returned to Doksat and fixed up accommodation
for the party, also calling for a strong partisan guard for the
village. The morale of the party was so low, I will not describe it. However, no incidents occurred and they accepted
my judgment and no effort was made to discuss the failure
further. Opened up with CAIRO and sent the following
message:

"Very regrettable a/c arrived to-day. Do not rpt not send
aircraft unless you receive all clear. Germans are now in
ARGYROKASTRON hence the absence of party on airfield
today. Self saw four MK IV tanks also troops. As it appears to
be just a looting expedition by Germans expect them to leave
any time. Propose staying here until all clear. Am now with
TILMAN who tried to send word of Germans as did self.
Grd signal will be five rpt five men on runway holding strips
of yellow parachute if no signal do not land. Operation flight
today perfect."

12   Marathon March

Report of Captain Lloyd G. Smith, OSS

30 December 1943

A later message dated December 30, 1943, instructed me to proceed according to the original plan. (At this time, I knew nothing about the attempt at air rescue.)

By this time (December 30, 1943) German activity around Dukati, Terbaci, Brataj, and Ramica was greatly reduced. Reports from our men stated that the Germans had withdrawn from most of the villages. This is SOP with the Germans. They move into a village, kill a few Partisans and after a few days, move out again.

I accordingly decided to move down into the Palasa-Dhermi area and to send out couriers on all possible routes to secure information as to the whereabouts of the party which was presumed to be making another attempt to reach the coast.

30 December 1943, Thursday—1015: Doksat

Refugees continued to come to Doksat and brought news of life in the city since the takeover. Some of the refugees described the American planes that had been seen the previous day, but they had no idea why the planes came.

Steffa visited, bringing the stories once or twice a day. "They said the Germans were frightened and taken totally by surprise. One man laughed as he told me about three German officers who were sitting and smoking cigars in a small tearoom where he worked. At the sound of the airplanes, the officers crawled, or tried to crawl under tables." Steffa laughed.

Jens was almost thoroughly convinced that they could have been rescued if only they had known ahead of time how many planes were being sent and how surprised the Germans would be by their arrival. She felt more sorry than ever for Gary. His decision must have been hard to make in the face of so much opposition. Jens never questioned him about it, and to the best of her knowledge, neither did anyone else.

Steffa was still pushing the idea that he could be of great help to the Allies if he were in Italy. "The pilots haven't said a flat 'no' to this proposition yet," he said.

"It isn't really their decision," Jens said. She hated getting drawn into the conversation, but Steffa always waited for a reply. "Gary is in ultimate charge. He only received the final word a day or so ago that *he* could leave the country with us. He probably has to okay whoever else goes with us. You saw for yourself yesterday that Gary has the final say on everything connected to getting us out of Albania."

"Yes, I saw. That was very highhanded on his part, don't you think?" Steffa waited for Jens's response.

"No, not really. If only they'd had time to verify the message, or if it had been clear. I believe his decision was difficult for him, with at least twenty-seven people pulling the opposite way, but that's his job, and frankly, I have a lot of faith in his ability. I felt very sorry for him when he had to face ten women with tears in their eyes. Gary has my total respect."

"But none of you three cried," Steffa said.

"We all shed a few tears," Elna said.

"Two of the girls are still crying today," Steffa said. "I know because I just visited them."

"Who? For heavens sake, if the planes are gone, they're gone! They'd better snap out of it," Marky said. Her voice was heavy with disgust.

After Steffa left, Jens decided to go upstairs to lie down.

"Don't even call me for food," she said. "Unless, of course, we should get steak, French fries, and salad. You know, that *best* meal!"

31 December 1943, Friday—0800:
Doksat to Saraginishte

For reasons unclear to Jens, Gary decided to move the party from Doksat to a village farther back from the coast. After a three-hour walk they arrived at Saraginishte, a cluster of five or six houses. When Jens and four other nurses arrived at the house assigned to them, their host was very busy loading what appeared to be a large trunk onto a horse-drawn, two-wheeled cart that stood at the entrance. After they were settled in, they looked out the small window on the opposite side of the house and saw a young man helping their host unload the trunk into a freshly dug hole in the earth. The men shoveled the dirt on top of it, carefully laying the sod in place and scattering a few rocks about the area.

"They don't seem to be in a hurry or especially excited, but I wonder why they're doing this today," Marky said.

Jean shrugged. "Maybe they just heard about the German occupation of Gjirokastër."

Lois, who usually played devil's advocate, said, "Or maybe the Germans are moving closer, and that's why we were asked to move from Doksat."

Marky groaned. "I should have known better than to think out loud beside you."

Lois giggled mischievously. "Just a pleasant thought for the last day of this year."

"That's right, it *is* New Year's Eve tonight!" Elna said.

The realization changed the subject from their present plight to reminiscences about previous New Year's Eves. They were interrupted when two women brought in a pot of stew with grease floating on top. As soon as Jens saw the grease, she felt nauseated and turned her back to the food; the sounds of the others' spoons hitting the side of the pot made her feel even sicker.

After supper they returned to recalling past New Year's Eve celebrations.

"Last year I was on call in the OR, and I was almost glad," Jens said. "I found it difficult to work up enthusiasm for a gala New Year's Eve in uniform." She laughed. "But things do change, don't they? This year I'd be happy just to have a *clean* uniform."

"I've never been an eggnog and fruitcake fan," Lois said, "but I sure would like to be at my mother's open house for New Year's Day."

Jens noticed that Elna was staring into the fire, oblivious to the conversation.

"What are you thinking about, Elna?" Jens asked.

Without looking at anyone, she said, "Home, and I don't mean Sicily. I mean way back home in South Dakota."

Jens suddenly remembered that while they were still at the port of embarkation in August, Elna had received a letter from her father with the news that her brother, a navy pilot, had been reported missing in action. There had been no further news from the Navy Department in any of the letters that she had received since.

Elna looked at Jens and smiled, "I can just smell my mother's cooking!"

Everyone sat quietly, and Jens figured that Elna knew she hadn't fooled anyone.

"Actually," Elna said, "I can't imagine a sadder place than home this New Year's Eve. By now they've probably received word that I'm missing too. It would have to make for a really sad holiday."

"Do you have other brothers and sisters?" Jean asked.

"Yes, I have a brother and sister, both younger. I know they'll be home with my parents, if they can get leave. My sister is a WAC and my brother's in the army."

Tooie looked at her watch. "It's only 8:30, but I can't think of one reason to wait up for 1944."

"Me neither," Jens said.

They settled around the fire, and in less than an hour, everyone was sound asleep.

Report of Lieutenant Gavin B. Duffy, SOE

[31 December 1943]

Received a signal on the 30th saying a/c came without our signal, but would continue to stand by.

Stayed at Doksat a further day, but decided to move to SARAGINISHTE for the following reasons:

1. To be nearer the exit up to SHEPR, in case the GERMANS came out to make trouble. It must be remembered I could see them from DOKSAT, moving on the road.
2. Shortage of food and general fear in the village. We were not exactly thrown out of the village, but ALBANIANS can be very passive! Very passive indeed!

On the move again! Back away from the coast. However, still in the vicinity of the airfield, but hoping desperately that the GERMANS would leave. Up to this time the GERMANS had not been particularly obstructive, though not very sociable from a humanitarian point of view!

Report of Captain Lloyd G. Smith, OSS

01 January 1944
On December 31, 1943, at 1000 hours, I left the base in the rain for sub-base at Grava Bay, arriving there at 1300 hours.

On New Years Day I left the sub-base at 1215 hours. It was still raining. At 1630 hours, I arrived at a shepherd's cave and decided to stay the night there.

02 January 1944, Sunday—1330: Saraginishte

Gary came in, sat in front of the fire, and chatted for fifteen minutes. The entire time, Jens felt sure he had something important to tell them.

"If the reports I'm receiving are correct," he finally said, "we'll be able to start again for the coast in a few days."

"You mean they've quit fighting?" Jens asked.

"They've stopped fighting," he said, "but the question now is whether the Germans have withdrawn completely or are occupying certain areas."

"Couldn't we skirt the areas they're in?" Lois asked.

Tight-lipped and exasperated, Gary answered curtly, "Perhaps, when we find out *where* those are!"

They got the message and didn't ask any more questions. He stood up to leave and motioned Jens to follow him.

"Jens, I need your opinion on a couple of things." She followed him out the door. "Some of the girls aren't at all well," he said. "Are you aware of that?"

"Yes. Actually, no one is totally well. We've been plagued with bouts of dysentery, some worse than others. Elna is quite jaundiced. Sergeant Cruise doesn't look at all well to me, but I don't know what's wrong with him. Sergeant Shumway's knee is better, but he's still limping. In a way, it doesn't really matter, because we have no more medicine." She paused and met Gary's eyes. "But who is ill today?"

"Well," he stammered and blushed, "there's a problem, or illness, with a few of the girls who say—well, they say that's why they're so cross and quarrelsome."

Still thinking about dysentery, hepatitis, and possible kidney infection, Jens said, "What illness are we talking about?"

He wrinkled his nose and scratched his head, looking at Jens as if she were terribly dense. Groping for words, he tried to spell it out for her. "Well, you know, each month something happens to girls—"

"Oh!" Jens felt as if a ton of bricks had fallen on her. "Oh, that!" She felt sure he was referring to the fact that most of the nurses had stopped menstruating after the first couple of weeks in Albania. Before she remembered to whom she was speaking, she said, "Well, me too, for that matter, but who has been telling you that's why they're cross and quarrelsome?" Before he could respond, she said, "Oh, never mind. I can guess. Gary, that's an excuse used by some women for their crossness, crying, or just about anything they don't want to take responsibility for—since time immemorial. All I can say is, I've never heard of anyone dying from it, and like everything else that's wrong with us right now there's not a darn thing we can do about it. Frankly, I consider it one of the few blessings on this jaunt!"

He looked so relieved, Jens thought for a moment he would break down and give her a kiss on the cheek. He didn't.

"Well, good, good!" he said quickly, inching away. "I really am quite hopeful we can leave here very soon!"

"Oh, I do hope so. If nothing else, there is less quarreling when we're on the move."

Jens wondered why any woman, especially a nurse, would confide in him about such problems.

Report of Lieutenant Gavin B. Duffy, SOE

[02 January 1944]
 After staying at SARAGINISHTE for two days during which time I had to settle financial accounts with the villagers (in which case I received a murderous 'hiding'), I decided to cancel the pick-up operation, for the following reasons. The weather had changed again, snow and heavy clouds; the GERMAN position, I could not guarantee. As I received a rather unfavourable report regarding the health of two of the nurses of the party from the Nurse in charge, I made a more concrete decision, and signaled CAIRO as follows:
"Ref pickup as GERMANS show no signs of evacuating GJINO and news that coast is clear have decided cancel planes and will proceed SEAVIEW. Will send THRASHER ahead so advise SMITH make contact KALARAT rpt KALARAT ETA 7th. Have made this decision in view uncertainty GERMAN ops this area."

Report of Captain Lloyd G. Smith, OSS

02 January 1944
 The following day (January 2, 1944), I left for Dhermi, arriving there at 1500 hours. Weather good.
 At Dhermi, I contacted an English-speaking friend and made arrangements for six men to start out in three different directions in search of information about the American party. The men were to travel in pairs and should the party be met, it was agreed that one of the two men should stay with the party, and the other should return to me with information. Two of the six men were to go to Terbaci; two to Vranishti and Kalarat and two to Kuc and Golem. These men all left Dhermi, the night of January 2, 1944.

03 January 1944, Monday—1630:
Saraginishte

Late the next afternoon Gary and the pilots came by to tell the nurses of consistent reports that the fighting had stopped and the Germans had left the area.

"I hope they are telling it straight for once, but at any rate, we shall start off tomorrow about 0800. I think I can get some mules for those who need to ride so we can move right along all day," Gary said in one long breath.

"How long do you think it might take us, if we can go straight through?" Elna turned her very jaundiced eyes to Gary. She was lying on her side by the fireplace. She remained cheerful but had seemed relieved to lie down by the fire any chance she could get during the past few days.

"Not more than a week, I'm sure!" he answered.

"And if we keep the mules with us, maybe we can make it in four or five days?" Tooie asked.

He shook his head and grinned. "You Americans are the eternal optimists!"

"Isn't that better than the other way around?" Jens asked.

He agreed immediately. "Oh, yes," he answered, then suddenly became very serious. "It's been nicer being with you because of your optimism, even with all our rotten luck so far!"

Jens felt he was referring to the planes specifically. She wanted to ask if he thought they might have made it had they been closer to the field and had he signaled the planes to land. She couldn't bring herself to ask the question.

04 January 1944, Tuesday—0730:
En Route to Kuc Once More

They left Saraginishte very early, racing along all day as though to make up for lost time. It had been dark for hours by the time that they reached the tiny village of Midhar. There were three houses and not a light in sight. Jens hoped no trigger-happy guards were about. One of the guides trotted ahead and arranged accommodations for the night at the first house he reached. The five or six people lying near the fireplace in the dingy room they entered merely moved over a space, pushing a sleeping baby goat or two along down the line to make room for the group. Jens was glad to sit down and pull off her shoes; she was relieved to find no blisters, despite the pace that Duffy had set all day. She barely nodded at the figures that rose on their elbows to look at them from across the fire or to greet them with a grin.

Jens lay down and would have been asleep in minutes if one of the baby goats hadn't decided to dance around playfully on her tired, aching feet. She pushed the kid away with her left foot, but it seemed to think that she was playing too and only became livelier. Fortunately, the woman across the fireplace heard the ruckus and grabbed the frolicsome goat by the nape of the neck, tucking him under her covers, and all was quiet again.

The entire party showed the ravages of constant dysentery and insufficient food, but they had vetoed any suggestions of stopping except for handouts and occasional rest. After so many reversals, they were obsessed with getting to the coast before anything else happened. "The coast" became the magic word for all kinds of help, especially rescue. It made little difference now how ill a person was, or with what sort of illness, since there was no more medicine. That fact became just one more reason to drive themselves constantly to reach their destination on the Adriatic Sea.

Gary seemed as eager to race on as any of them. Perhaps an added impetus for him was that his latest orders were to leave the country with the Americans.

Report of Gavin B. Duffy, SOE

[05 January 1944]
MIDHAR TO GOLEM, M.21
My next halt was GOLEM, a village with only 7 or 8 houses left standing. THRASHER had gone ahead to arrange food, shelter, etc. The weather, after leaving MIDHAR was treacherous—rain and violent hailstorms. About one hour from GOLEM, I thought several of the girls were going

to crack up, I myself being almost on the point of doing so, so I set the pace for a while, kept dropping in the rear—in fact, I literally pushed them through. We arrived GOLEM amidst hail and snow, looking like a bunch of prisoners on the Russian front. The party, within an hour, were distributed to various homes.

The following message was sent from GOLEM the same night:—

"Party now at GOLEM M.2912. Am pushing party through day and night. Please ensure little delay as possible at SEASIDE as party having rough time this area. May reach KALARAT M. 1319 tomorrow."

Report of Captain Lloyd G. Smith, OSS

05 January 1944
That night (January 5, 1944) I left on a truck with some Partisans, arriving at Vuno at 2100 hours.

05 January 1944, Wednesday—1530:
To Kuc via Golem

The day suddenly turned gloomy, damp, and cold. Jens hoped it wouldn't snow. It didn't, but the sleet, along with a driving wind in their faces, was much worse than snow. Her weather-beaten trench coat soon became soaked through, and her shoulders and feet ached with the wet and cold. They slipped and slid along; only the little mules seemed surefooted. They gave up about 1600 hours, when they reached a small hamlet that Jens recognized immediately. They were in Golem again—for the third time—and each time it had rained or sleeted, or hailed. This time they were subjected to a mixture of the three. Fortunately, this time, the people decided to take them in for the night.

Report of Lieutenant Gavin B. Duffy, SOE

[06 January 1944]
During the night, a very heavy snow had fallen. My first

glimpse in the morning was ground depth 2" snow and more falling. To acquire mules from this village was impossible. Having collected the party together, I informed them it was going to be a rough trip and asked them if they were ready. "Aye, Mr. Gary," they replied, "let's get hoofing!" Then Miss Jensen, the senior nurse informed me that Miss Tacina had a bad ankle. On inspection, I found it swollen. She protested vigorously, saying it was "O.K., swell!" Feeling, of course, that she may hold the party back. I knew she could not walk more than 100 yards, and as expected, she started up the hill and after 50 yards, she collapsed. I was behind her. I then had to hail the party in front, but owing to the blizzard, they could not hear me. With the aid of Miss Jensen, another nurse and Sgt. BELL, I dumped some of our personal kit, overloading the other three mules, which was to prove fatal, and managed to put Miss Tacina on a mule. We carried on, but after two hours, the guide, bless him, lost the way for about half an hour. You could not see a hand in front of you. The guide was scared and wished to stay on top of the mountain and wait until the blizzard cleared. For the first time, I lost my temper and nearly strangled him; at the same time, my interpreter conveyed verbally, my wish. We then set off again and after an hour, passed out of the blizzard.

How those girls took it, I do not know. We were going in the direction of KUC, down the hill into the valley, when the mule Miss Tacina was riding, stumbled. I had been holding the mule's tail, going down, when over the side of the mule she went. Below her was a gradual drop of about 15 feet. I made a headlong dive after her, just catching hold of her belt and we both rolled down the hill together, emerging from the drift, just two huge snow balls! Luckily, neither of us was hurt.

Back on the mule and away again. The mules had no food for two days and were cracking up. Later on, a further mule went down carrying the batteries. This stayed down for half an hour, but did rise and carry on later, groaning all the while—most reassuring!

Pushing on, we reached KUC. To sleep there was practically impossible. We decided to carry on, gaining by now, two and a half days. Leaving Kuc, it was necessary to cross a tributary of the Shushicë to get on a second class road for KALARAT. Here a further incident occurred.

The men, in order to ford this fast and deep stream, used poles and vaulted across. The girls hardly had the strength to lean! As I was wearing rubber boots, I stood in the center of the stream, water round my thighs and assisted the girls across—it could hardly be called assisted! I just slung them across. Everything during this acrobatic display was going fine, until the last nurse produced a bit more energy than the others, and came at me like a tornado. Down I went backwards, in the stream, receiving, as you can well imagine, a substantial drenching. She fared quite well. This day of incidents! Not amusing at the time though!

About an hour away from our destination, I saw coming towards us a bearded foreigner, obviously so, as ALBANIANS do not wear beards. Halting when he reached us, he informed us he was Capt. SMITH. The name SMITH struck a familiar chord!

13 The American Captain Smith

06 January 1944, Thursday—1400: En Route to KALARAT

When Jens stepped off the trail to rest, straighten her shoulders, stretch her aching back, and wiggle her aching toes, three figures approached them and began shouting something to Gary, who was somewhere behind her. As Jens strained to see the three more clearly, Allen shouted, "My God, it's Smith. Captain Smith, that is!" He and three other sergeants ran up to Smith, gave a halfhearted salute, and gripped his hand.

Sergeant Allen said, "You don't know how good you look to us. Even those railroad tracks are a sight for sore eyes!"

Captain Lloyd Smith, the long-awaited American OSS man, had come walking jauntily along, swinging a stick, and accompanied by two Albanians. His cap, captain's bars, and paratrooper's boots were the only American parts of his uniform. He wore a heavy wool British battle jacket, trousers tucked inside his boots, and an Albanian cape of black, coarse wool folded back over his shoulders. He was of average height, with a blond beard and mustache.

"This is a nice surprise," Smith said. "I really didn't expect to run into you for at least another day. What day did you actually start?"

"The fourth as planned," Gary spoke up. He grinned a little. "We have been making very good time!"

"You sure have." Smith looked around the group. They gathered in close, just to hear another American voice.

"We were really expecting to meet you about the fifteenth or sixteenth of December," Jens said. "Then we got word that you'd been captured."

"Yeah, well I got some of those stories about you too," Smith said. "I don't know where these people get all that glum news, but they seemed to hike in from a fair distance just to impart it."

Gary shook his head. "You just can't believe a word they say. Out of every six reports, you pick one and hope you chose right, but it's better to check for yourself when you can."

Smith walked down the trail, flanked by the pilots who talked a blue streak to him. He talked to the stragglers, heard their complaints, and moved them to the front of the line so they could set the pace for everyone.

That night, as they sat around a fireplace in Kalarat, Smith peppered them with questions on how they had managed for almost two months since the crash landing.

"You've certainly done well for yourselves," he said. "You must have followed Gary's instructions pretty well."

"We certainly did," Jens said. "I'm not sure where we'd be now if we hadn't had him as a leader."

"How about the three nurses who are missing? When did you last hear from them?"

"We haven't. That's just it," Jens said. "Most of us feel they must still be in Berat. Someone must be hiding them. I guess you know that the Germans have occupied the town. We've been told by villagers that whenever the Germans ask questions about us, they describe us as a large American party that includes thirteen nurses. We thought that was a good indication that they haven't been picked up yet, and if they'd gotten out of Berat safely, surely we would have heard by now." She nodded toward Gary. "He doesn't believe they're POWs either."

Smith looked at Gary, "Why?"

"Unless the Germans have changed their tactics, they're more inclined to spout that kind of news than we are, and there hasn't been a word from anywhere. They haven't even spun any fairytales about them."

Smith smiled and nodded thoughtfully. "They must be lying low somewhere, most likely in Berat."

"How can we reach them there?" Jens asked. "They won't have to stay there until the end of the war, will they?"

"There are ways of contacting them, and even sending a vehicle in with the right stickers and passes to get them by all the checkpoints."

Lois laughed. "Wouldn't that beat all, if they get a ride to the coast while we have climbed, slipped, and slid all over this country for sixty days?"

Two Albanians came into the room and motioned to Smith. He spoke with them and returned to the party ten minutes later.

"We have a little good news," Smith said. "I've just received word that the Germans have left Terbaci. That means we can take a more direct route."

"What would we have done if they were still in town?" Jens asked.

"We could have gone over the mountains to a cave southwest of Palasa. I've already stored emergency rations in the cave, just in case we had to go that way. It would take four days to reach the Base by that route, and we wouldn't be able to use the mules."

"I'm very glad the Germans pulled out," Jens said.

"Aren't we all!" Tooie said. "Aren't we all!"

07 January 1944, Friday—0815: En Route to Terbaci and Dukat

The group gathered in the morning cold to wait for Smith and Gary. Jens spotted Steffa walking toward her. He extended his right hand, and she took it automatically.

"I'm going back now," Steffa said. "I can't travel any farther into Ballist territory." His eyes were filling with tears.

Without thinking, Jens blurted out, "You aren't going to the coast with us?"

"No," he said. "Germans and Ballista are too concentrated throughout the area. I'll be going back alone."

"I'm sorry," Jens said simply. She felt sick, despite all the doubts the group had shared concerning Steffa's loyalties.

"You remember I told you I have two brothers in Cleveland, Ohio?"

"Yes, I remember."

"Please write them when you return to Italy. I'm asking you because you stayed at my house and met all my family, and my elderly parents. Please tell them about us, just how you saw us. We are well and get along pretty good in spite of everything. They have inquired through the Red Cross several times, but I'm sure they don't hear much more than that we're alive."

"Of course, I'll write to your brothers," Jens promised. "I still remember playing a game of cards with your mother. It was one of the more pleasant evenings we spent in Albania."

"Thank you. Thank you," he smiled through his tears.

While they were talking, Jens had removed her flight wings and was holding them in her hand. Many times she'd started to give them to Steffa for his eldest son. The first time they met, the boy had admired them and asked excitedly, mainly through sign language, if Jens were a pilot. As long as Steffa was with the Americans, however, she had felt it better to keep them herself, in case they were ambushed or captured. She handed them to him now. "I'd like your son to have these, unless you'd rather not carry them now."

He took them quietly and wiped a tear away. "He'll be very pleased. I remember how excited he was because he thought you were a pilot." They laughed together.

Suddenly, he grabbed her hand again. "Goodbye. I must tell the others goodbye too. I wish you a safe trip to Italy."

"Thank you," Jens said. "Thank you for everything. Goodbye." The words sounded silly and stupid to her. They seemed so little to say to one who had been their means of food and shelter and communication in all kinds of weather and circumstances. Maybe he had a selfish reason for doing all this, but they had an equally selfish one—to stay alive.

Jens looked about and listened to other goodbyes. Panda was turning back too, and two of the guides had decided to go no farther. Who's going to show us the way, Jens wondered. She was relieved to see two other Albanians in the crowd, in addition to the two who were traveling with Smith.

They were soon in their long line again, following the guides and mules. Several of the party stopped to look back at Steffa and Panda, who were watching from a small bluff. They waved, and the Americans waved back. They turned and walked into the distance as the group watched them disappear beyond the mountain.

Jens took the slip of paper Steffa had given her out of her pocket. It read: "Telemak Steffa, George Steffa, 29th Street, Cleveland, O." She wrote George's number down on her diary, along the edge of a column, and the street on another page. She knew she would never forget the name Steffa, and felt sure she'd remember the name George. She tore Steffa's paper into tiny bits, letting the pieces fly in the wind as she walked along the trail.

They stopped for a quick lunch arranged by Thrasher and an interpreter, whom Smith had sent on ahead to Terbaci. In forty minutes they were on the trail again. It was 1500 when they approached a cluster of four houses.

"Let's stop here, get some food, rest a while, and talk over our situation," Smith said. He was so calm and matter of fact that Jens's confidence in him had gone sky high. She felt completely relaxed, questioned nothing he said, and only waited to hear his next decision. Gary and the pilots seemed to have given him free reign, and all discord had suddenly evaporated. She also suspected that they were all too exhausted to raise a voice in dissent any longer.

As they approached the first house, a man came out on the porch. Before they could speak a word, he quickly told them how much he'd like to help, but the Germans had taken everything in their sweep through there a few weeks earlier. "They took all our chickens," Smith's interpreter said. Just then three happy, healthy hens came strolling cautiously by. The Albanian looked at them from the corner of his eye and mumbled something. The interpreter went right on. "He says they must be the neighbor's." Two goats tied under a tree by the house began to bleat their presence too.

Captain Smith had evidently decided to stop and wasn't about to be deterred. He stepped up to the interpreter who was pleading the man's case.

"Tell him to go ask his neighbors to help put something together to feed us. We must have some food before we can go on. I have money to pay for the meal and their trouble, and also we'd like to come inside to wait and sit down for a while."

The man stared at Smith for a few seconds, and Smith met his eyes. Then the villager stepped back, opened the door, and nodded for them to enter. Squatting on the floor, they waited quietly to hear what Smith had on his mind. He outlined the situation to them without preliminaries.

"The rest of the way has to be traveled at night. We have only one choice: we stay right here tonight and all day tomorrow, or we leave here this evening, after a couple hours of rest, and continue to the coast."

There was a chorus of voices, all with the same message. "Let's leave today. We can't sit here a whole day just waiting for darkness."

Smith looked surprised, but pleased. "You're sure you can go on today? You've been pushing mighty hard the past few days as it is."

"We can go on," Jean said. "Everything has been going good so far. Let's keep it going."

Everyone agreed except Thrasher. "It's up to the girls," he said, pushing the decision onto the women. "If they can take it, we can."

The nurses were furious. "What do you mean, if the girls can take it! We've been on our feet all the way, haven't we? And who has been taking care of all of you when you got sick?" Jens asked.

Thrasher cringed and looked to Smith for help.

"I say let's go on tonight," Lois said quickly during the brief lull, just in case the decision hadn't been clinched yet.

Sergeant Zeiber spoke up. "Sir, it's my opinion that these gals will make it in good shape, and if we are that close, let's make a dash for it."

Smith was silent.

"I can't see that Adriatic soon enough!" Tooie said.

When things quieted down, Smith said, "Well, okay, we'll go on tonight. But once we start, we can't stop. We *must* make it over the last ridge and out of sight by daybreak tomorrow."

"I hope we can still have mules to carry our sick people and some of our junk," Jens said.

"We will," Smith answered.

"Gee, if I were sure we'd make it, I'd give away my musette bag and everything in it right now."

Smith said, "We'll have mules."

Food finally arrived. They evidently had to bake a few wheels of cornbread for the mob. It was warm, and it smelled good. Jens sat with a large chunk of the pungent, white goat's milk cheese. "You know, I've sort of developed a taste for this stuff."

Smith got up to leave. "Finish your food," he said. "It will take a while to get ready." Gary, the pilots, and some of the men followed him out.

The couple of hours they were given to rest was anything but peaceful. As Jens stepped out onto the porch, she could hear loud voices. Two Albanians were shouting back and forth. Smith stood beside them with his interpreter, as well as Gary and Blondie. In the center of the group were three mules with their heads hanging down, acting as if they wanted to doze if only the men would be quiet.

Smith patted his interpreter on the back and stated quietly and firmly, "You ask him how much the mules are worth. I'll buy them. With *gold*," he emphasized.

The answer came back, "No, he doesn't want to sell his mules because, he says, he can't buy more."

Smith insisted. "I'll pay for the mules and you can still have them when we're finished with them tonight. What more could you ask?"

The man seemed doubtful that anyone would bring them back to him. Jens wanted to see the gold that Smith seemed to have in his hand. She visualized gold nuggets, but they sounded like coins. As he jingled them, the man remained adamant and tried to grab his mules. Smith laid the money down on the edge of the porch and pulled out his gun. He didn't point it, but looking straight into the reluctant villager's terrified eyes he said, "Just tell him I'm taking the mules. We've got to have them for tonight. I hope he can find some-one to bring them back to him or he can come along with us."

He stood and waited a minute for the interpreter to translate. The frightened man looked limp as he nodded and glanced at the money. Smith turned around and said, "Everybody ready? Let's hit the trail."

It was a little after 1700. Jens heard Smith and the pilots discussing the latest episode. "I wasn't sure that would work, but one way or another, I wasn't leaving without the mules."

"He didn't come, did he?" Thrasher asked as he peered over his shoulder.

"No," the interpreter said. "He is too afraid of the Ballista through here. He wants me to arrange for their return when we are finished."

"Well, I hope they get back to him," Smith said.

In an hour they were in snow, which got deeper as they continued climbing. The whole area was beautiful, with not a track in it but theirs. However, the snow made walking treacherous and exhausting. The mules were ahead of them, breaking a path. Eventually, they were in belly deep and couldn't get their little short legs up over the heavy snow piles. The riders jumped off to permit the animals to go forward. The mule carrying the nurses' coats and bags fell onto its knees. They tried to coax him up, but he seemed more inclined to lie there and rest for a while.

"Let's unload him before he decides to spend the night," Jens suggested. The women grabbed their coats, put them on and each one took a musette bag or some piece of gear. They kicked at the mule and pulled his tail until he finally got up and followed the others.

"Well, at least they can break a trail for us," Sergeant Owen said.

"Yeah, and if they slide over the side, we will at least know to hug the opposite side a little more." Sergeant Zeiber had been a continuous source of this kind of black humor.

Jens hadn't seen Smith all evening and learned that he had struck out ahead. A full moon rose well up in the sky behind them, dispelling some of the darkness. As one mule after another collapsed in snow that was just too deep for them, some of the taller men went out ahead to help break a path. This is ridiculous, Jens thought. These mules had better get some rest or no one will be able to ride them downhill. Tired of carrying her musette bag, she pulled out her mess kit and a shirt and asked the guide ahead of her if anyone might want the mess kit. He reached out for it, saying that he would like to have it. She decided to hand him the whole bag so he could keep whatever he wanted. I'm sure we'll make it this time, she reasoned. If not— tough! She now had only the clothes on her back and realized that the few possessions that had meant so much to her were suddenly worthless.

As they neared the top of the mountain the snow wasn't nearly so deep, and they began to see evergreens, a rarity in Albania. As tired as Jens was, she could still appreciate the beautiful, clear, crisp night. She stopped and looked around, recalling many identical nights of moonlight when, as a kid, she had gone sledding in Michigan. This long sloping hill would be ideal for that old bobsled they'd had so much fun with; it could have gone all the way down to the bottom in record time unless the snow was too deep. She remembered times when it piled right into the snow but its riders kept right on going, end over end, down the hill. She hadn't seen a sled of any kind in Albania, or anything for children to have a little fun with, and she was struck by the grimness of the country.

At the bottom of the trail a dozen or two houses, nestled among a few tall trees, were scattered along a wide dirt street. They seemed better built than most they had seen in Albania. Some had tall columns supporting a roof over a small front door step, reminiscent of the colonial style in America.

This was Dukat, by far the most pleasant town they had seen in the country. It looked neat, clean, and bright in the moonlight. Smith and Gary stood waiting for them under a clump of trees, and they were ushered into several houses as though they were expected.

The ten nurses were assigned to a house that was nicely furnished with a few comfortable chairs, and a huge leather hassock in front of a big fireplace with a roaring fire. Their hosts brought them a tea tray, complete with a sugar bowl. Jean cautiously peeked into it and found that it contained coarse sugar. *Sugar*! A whole bowl full! Where did they get sugar, Jens wondered. Although she did not ordinarily take sugar, she put a big spoonful into her tea, and it never tasted better. There were crackerlike cakes, the inevitable goat's milk cheese, another cheese she had never seen before, and cornbread that actually tasted good.

The two Albanian women in the room, dressed in western-style skirts and sweaters, tried to make polite conversation in Albanian. Jens did a mental inventory of the room and decided they were living better than anyone else she had seen in the country. These women had sugar, salt, and leavening agents, all of which, Steffa had told them earlier, had to be imported. There seemed only one possibility to Jens; they had to be friends of the Germans or Ballista. But then why were they helping the Americans? Had Smith ordered this too? If they weren't friends of the Germans, they must be making a good pretense of it; otherwise why would they be left alone with more material wealth than anyone else she had seen in Albania? Jens glanced at her watch and was even more curious about the women being so prepared to offer them their hospitality—it was ten minutes before midnight.

After they finished their late lunch, they sat around getting warm and drowsy, waiting for word from Smith.

08 January 1944, Saturday—0130: Dukat to the Coast

Shortly after 0130 there was a knock on the door. The younger woman scurried to open it, and after exchanging only a few words with the caller she motioned for the nurses to leave. They shook hands, thanked their hosts, and filed out. A man led them quickly down the dirt street for a block or two, where the rest of the group had assembled behind a small army truck. Jens was startled at first and couldn't decide whether the truck was good or bad news. Smith motioned for them to come closer.

"We're going to ride this truck for a ways," he said. "It will save at least four hours of walking, but we'll have to be careful, so listen up." Smith's face was half in moonlight, half in shadow. "If we meet any vehicle on the road, we have to assume that it's German. Our truck will stop, and everybody must get off as quickly as possible. Get off the truck and get as far from it as you can. You girls and unarmed men, take cover, lie flat, and be quiet. Only the driver stays with the truck. He'll pretend to have motor trouble. If they get too nosy and insistent, we'll just have to dispose of them."

He looked over at Gary, and Jens followed his glance to Blondie,

Bert, a British soldier from Seaview, and his interpreter. They all had guns slung across their shoulders. He motioned with his hands for emphasis. "There would probably be three or four of them in a car, so we can't fool around if their suspicions are aroused." He looked from face to face. "Any questions?" No one spoke. "Okay then. Let's get going."

It was 0200. Jens wondered where Smith had collected all this equipment on such short notice. Clearly gold was magic! They climbed on board in silence. Smith and Gary sat in front with the driver, while the rest of the group crammed into the back, several sitting on the floor. Blondie and Bert stood in the back, clinging to the canopy. There was scarcely room for a deep breath. The truck jerked to a start and had barely got rolling when it made a sharp turn, leaving the town behind them, and headed down a hard, rough dirt road. Surrounded by others, Jens couldn't see a thing, and the canopy closed out the moonlight entirely. Not a word was spoken as they bumped and rumbled along, the truck swaying back and forth as it took the turns along a mountain road.

Suddenly they stopped so abruptly that people were thrown forward against each other. Smith was at the back of the truck before anyone could move.

"Get out! Get out—hurry up! A car's coming! Get behind those rocks over there," he shouted.

Jens leaped straight off the end of the truck and ran toward the huge boulders she could see a short distance from the road. Just before she reached the first boulder, she caught her toe under a tough, creeping vine and pitched headlong. As she lay there, dazed and moaning, someone came along behind her and gave her a poke in the back. "Are you all right?"

She raised her head, so dazed that for several seconds, she couldn't speak. "Yeah, yeah. I'm all right," she finally mumbled.

"Well, get up then, and get going," Sergeant Allen said.

She leaped up, ran, and dropped behind the first boulder she came to. There wasn't a sound, and she could barely see the truck and the driver in front of it. Where was the car that had routed them? Seconds later its headlights flashed around a sharp turn. The car slowed down and came to a stop beside their truck. Jens couldn't see anything but headlights until two men came into view, beside the driver. They talked for barely a minute, then headed back to their vehicle. The driver slammed the hood down as the men drove off. No one moved until Smith appeared beside the truck, waved, and called quietly to them. As they scrambled out from behind the boulders and climbed back on the truck, Smith said, "Okay. We were lucky this time. They were Germans, but they weren't curious tonight."

They careened around sharp turns and bumped along faster than before, as if trying to make up lost time. Suddenly the truck slid to a stop so fast that Jens hardly had time to think of the reason. The men with guns leaped off and ran. Then Smith appeared. "Run for cover—that way." He pointed to the left side of the road. "Hurry, duck out of sight. They're right on us this time."

As Jens raced across the road, she could see the glare of the ominous headlights coming up a hill, a little ahead of them. The ground was covered with those low, creeping bushes loaded with thorns, a menace of Albania that she had come to hate. The thorns grabbed hold of her slacks. The more she tried to push through the vines, the more places they took hold. She couldn't pull loose, so she dropped down into the vines, as deep and flat as possible. Jens felt someone drop down close to her. In just two seconds she knew who it was. Pauleen was cursing a blue streak. "Those G.D. elephants have no manners. Just stomped all over me until I couldn't get up or move. Next time, I'll let the SOBs go and just stay on the truck."

"Can we depend on that?" Jens heard a loud male stage whisper to her left.

Jens almost laughed, but headlights flashed down the road, and she could see the vehicle, a small pickup truck, as it rolled to a stop. Slowly she made out the silhouette of three men by the vehicle. Two of them talked to the Americans' driver, and from a word or two Jens could hear she felt sure they were Albanians. Finally they returned to their vehicle and left. The driver looked right and left, then signaled the group to return.

The next stop was slow and gentle, and Jens was glad to be told they were to leave the truck and the road. In the dark they picked their way through the brush for a few hundred feet until they came to a small house. The room they entered was lit by a dim lantern, standing on a box in one corner, and warmed by a potbellied stove. She sat down in a straight-backed chair beside the stove and promptly went to sleep.

It was 0430 when Jean poked Jens and said, "Come on. We're going."

As she got up to follow, she noticed that two British officers whom she had not met before, were standing in a nearby doorway, but she was too exhausted to be curious about them—from the base, she thought. She merely said, "Hi," and staggered after the tail end of the column that was fast disappearing through the back door.

The moon had disappeared, and there was no discernible trail. They just started up the side of the mountain in front of them, hoping for the best. She could see only those closest around her. Scrambling over rocks and low scrub to keep up, it seemed to her she slipped back one step for every two forward. Others were advancing at about the same rate.

As the first faint light of morning appeared, Jens could see the top of the ridge outlined against the sky and remembered that they had all promised Smith they would be on the other side of the ridge before daylight. Yet the more she tried to hurry, the more she slipped or stumbled, so finally she resigned herself to a steady, careful pace, glancing ahead only to make sure she was on the right track. She was so tired she felt sure that if she allowed herself to stop and lie down for a second, she would fall fast asleep.

When Gary, Smith, and Blondie came to the rear to gather up the stragglers, Jens was surprised to learn that there were some behind her. She heard Gary say, "I guess it's safe to send him on ahead with the message now."

Jens asked, "What message?"

"To tell the fellows down at the cave to wire for the boat to come to pick us up."

"Oh," Jens said, but she was too tired to realize the import of Gary's words.

At full daylight, not even half the party was at the top of the ridge. Blondie passed Jens as he led three mules down to pick up some of the slowest and get them over the top.

Jens stopped to catch her breath and look back over the territory they had just covered. The view was magnificent! A small pen-
insula extended into the sea many feet below them. She could see an
airstrip where a few small planes appeared to be taking off, circling
the field, and landing in a very short pattern. They must be practic-
ing, Jens thought, and of course they had to be German. She now
understood why they had to get over the last ridge and out of sight:
too much activity up there might well attract attention. She pushed
herself to climb the last hundred feet and found another beautiful
view spread out before her. Far below and as far as the eye could see
was the beautiful Adriatic. She walked down the opposite side several feet, and sat down to drink in the longed-for sight.

"We made it! I knew we could. I just knew we'd make it!" Jens
looked around for the source of the voice and realized it was her
own. Her eyes came back to the barren land at the edge of the sea,
and followed it back up the mountain to where she sat. It wasn't
nearly as steep as the side they'd climbed, but it would be a long
hike to wherever that cave Gary had mentioned might be. The
hillside was full of people; their group seemed to have grown overnight. Several more British from the base had apparently joined
them at some point. Now she no longer felt alone as she sometimes had while they traveled in the darkness of the long, exhausting night.

Report of Captain Lloyd G. Smith, OSS

08 January 1944
    The "safe house" was reached at 0345 hours. Here we
secured fresh mules, and the party started up the mountain
towards the Base at 0500 hours. It was necessary to reach a
point high on the mountain before daylight, in order that
the Germans could not spot us from the highway. The
summit of the mountain was reached at 0930 hours and a
message was dispatched to the Base via a shepherd. This
message requested that preparations be made for receiving
the party and suggested also that evacuation be arranged for
that night.

08 January 1944, Saturday—1015:
Descent from the Last Mountain

Several British officers climbed up to introduce themselves and shake the hands of the Americans.

"Welcome to this side of the mountain! We've been waiting a long time for you!"

Jens had been sitting on a rock for at least twenty minutes when she saw a British major climbing toward them with long springing steps. As he got closer, Jens could see that he was handing something to each person he met. When he reached Sergeant Allen, she knew exactly what it was. Allen let out a war whoop. "Hot damn! I knew if I made it, someone would hand me a pack of cigs! And by damn, they're even my brand." He tossed a pack of Philip Morris above his head and caught it as it came down.

Jens sat on the rock and savored each little morsel of the Hershey bar the major gave her. She couldn't remember when anything had tasted so good. All the rest of the way down the mountain her tongue searched around her teeth and occasionally found the thinnest of particles hiding there. Each time it was hard to realize that such a minute piece could have so much flavor.

It was nearly 1300 before Jens staggered to the level area at the entrance of the cave, a gaping hole in the side of the hill. Others were already there, gathered around a British captain who sat on a high stump, facing a two-burner Coleman stove. He had a chicken boiling in one pot, and into a frying pan on the other burner he plopped an egg for each newcomer. He was a most cheerful chef, and Jens would have sworn, as she peeled an orange and watched him, that there was nothing he'd rather be doing. She smiled and spoke to him.

"The only other orange I had before in this country I ate with the peel on, just like an apple. I remember it was very good."

Even the little bit of grease he used for the eggs nauseated her, however, so she took a cup of chicken broth instead. She was wondering what was holding her up, when the Captain pointed to the entrance and said, "There are bunks in there, so why not go lie down for a spell?"

She climbed up on the shiny, dark gray rock that was the floor of the cave and half-crawled the rest of the way into the interior. In the dim light cast by a few lanterns she could make out eight or ten bunks lined up side by side, and she collapsed beside other nurses who were already sacked out. The cave was much larger than she had imagined. A makeshift desk of rough-hewn wood with a small stool stood near the entrance and held one of the lanterns. The pilots and two British lay on bunks near her, exchanging tales of their harrowing experiences in Albania. She tried to listen but soon was sound asleep. The next thing she knew, someone was poking her.

"Jens, Jensen, wake up. Come on, get up!" Jean said.

Always get up and get going, she thought. She had half a mind to roll over and go back to sleep until a more insistent nudge came. "Come on, the boat is here!"

"The boat! Oh, that's right, the boat!" Jens grabbed her shoes and coat and struck out after the others. They were led down through a tangle of brush to the water's edge where she could see the dark silhouette of a boat, well off shore.

"Where are the others?" Jens asked in a half-whisper.

"Two loads have gone out already," Sergeant Allen said.

"What time is it? Do you know?" Jens asked.

"About midnight," Jean said.

A large rowboat slid quietly to shore in front of them. Jens and four others got in, and three men pushed it out just as quietly, jumping in as it was rowed away from the land. As they came alongside the larger boat, a man in a black overcoat stood up and grabbed a rope ladder, pulling it into the rowboat. Jens was closest to the ladder. The man handed it to her and said in English, "Crawl up. Hold the ropes tight!"

The boat pitched constantly, making the climb difficult, but before she got all the way to the top two men reached down, siezed her arms, and hauled her up. As she scrambled for her footing the two men, never releasing their vice-like grip marched her between them across the unlighted deck, through a blackout curtain, and down four steps. Jens couldn't imagine why they had held her so tight until one of them said, "Can you walk okay?"

"Sure," she said. "Why not?"

"We're just surprised to find you all on your feet."

They let go of her and rushed back up the stairs. Jens walked through a narrow passageway toward a lighted room. She looked inside. A bathroom at last! Marky was sitting on the floor, hugging the porcelain commode.

"Are you hurt?" Jens asked. "Did you fall?"

"No. I'm just seasick from this pitching boat."

Jens extended her hand. "Here, I'll help you up."

"No, just leave me here. I'll sleep beside this commode."

"Well, I wanted to use it," Jens said.

"Go ahead," Marky said. "Isn't it beautiful? So *white*!"

When she left Marky, Jens went into the officers' quarters, where there were two sets of double-deck bunks. All but one already had two occupants apiece. She peeled off her shoes, coat, and jacket and lay down on the empty one. Someone crawled in beside her, but she fell asleep without bothering to find out who it was.

An overhead light was shining on her face when she awakened. Others were up and moving about as she heard, "Breakfast is being served." Hot coffee was all Jens could think of. When she reached the galley, a familiar voice behind the counter made her look beyond the bowl being offered to her. It was Elna, smiling happily.

"We made some nice hot oatmeal with cold, canned sliced peaches!" Her grin went from ear to ear.

"We're certainly glad to have all of you on board, finally," a member of the boat's crew said to the group of four who were seated at a small table.

"It sounds as if you've been expecting us for some time," Jens said.

"You might say that," the young man answered. "They held us in port at Bari for almost a month, waiting for the message we received yesterday."

The thought that the military had held a boat in port, waiting to pick them up, surprised Jens and filled her with deep pride in being part of the Allied Forces fighting Hitler. She thought again of the grassy airfield at Gjirokastër, where eighteen P-38s, two C-47s, and a Wellington bomber had circled with the sole mission of bringing her group back to Allied territory. Even now the memory brought goose bumps to her skin and a lump to her throat. How wonderful to be part of an organization that valued each individual life so highly, an organization whose members would risk their lives gladly to rescue a downed comrade.

At 1355 on 9 January 1944, two months after they had flown out of Sicily to pick up wounded GIs, the boat carrying ten army nurses, thirteen army technical sergeants, and the air crew of four, pulled into port at Bari, Italy. Among the crowd waiting to greet them was their commanding officer. As they disembarked, they waved at him.

"Are we still in the army, Major?" Jens called.

Report of Lieutenant Gavin B. Duffy, SOE

09 January 1944

We had to leave here and start to climb in darkness and before day break "just over the top." Looking at the map, this "over the top" measures about 1". This in actual fact took eight hours. About two hours from Seaview, we could view the sea in all its glory! I left the party at this point and pushed ahead to the HQ to send a message as follows:

"From Duffy. Arrived with party SEAVIEW. All party completely worn out but morale high."

After eating, Commander Glen informed us that a boat was coming that evening. Most of the party fell asleep; others carried on eating.

These last four days had certainly been hectic. During this period, the party had slept for only eight hours. The boat did arrive and without even a glance back at the land, the party crawled aboard an M.I. bound for BARI.

We drew in at the port and received quite a reception. Dozens of official army photographers and a fleet of brand new cars were there to meet us. The Americans entered the staff cars and Sgt. BELL and myself were escorted to a G.S. 15 cwt. We were then taken to our HQ BARI, under the supervision of Capt. WATROUS, and the Americans were taken to a hospital under the care of "A" Force.

09 January 1944, Sunday—1545:
Twenty-sixth General Hospital, Bari

Immediately upon their arrival in Bari, they were whisked off to the Twenty-sixth General Hospital in staff cars. Before they could bathe or shed their lice-ridden clothes they were interrogated, individually and in groups. The major who questioned Jens was especially interested in what towns they had been in, who had helped them, whether the Germans had been a great threat, and how they had been able to manage without knowing the language.

Jens told him of the Albanians who had learned their English at the American-Albanian vocational school operated by the American Red Cross. She told the major that they all had spoken highly of a Mr. Harry Fultz, who had been the headmaster and principal teacher there about ten or fifteen years earlier. Their admiration for him knew no bounds, as they spoke of how he had taught them not only English but a great deal about the United States as well.

The major merely nodded as she talked, but then said, "As long as you are in this theater, don't mention his name again."

Jens immediately thought, he's probably serving our country right here in Italy. In fact, as she found out after the war, he had been serving as a primary consultant for Albanian affairs for the OSS Albanian desk at Bari.

To help herself recall the exact villages they were in at various times, Jens pulled her diary from her jacket pocket, but as she folded the papers to put them back, the major reached for them, saying, "I'll have to take those."

"Oh, no!" she said.

He assured her that she could write to the Prisoner of War Department in Washington after the war, and they would be sent to her. Jens was pleasantly surprised when, years later, she requested and received her diary.

Jens knew she was too exhausted at the time of her interview to appreciate fully the impact of it all. Rescue, finally. Food and shelter could again be taken for granted. But at that moment, she couldn't take her eyes off the clean, painted white walls!

Then came the luxury of a warm bath to soak in and scrub. A

little yellow pimple on her left calf didn't seem significant as she scrubbed over it, but hours later that area of her leg was sore and inflamed. She was given sulfa and warm soaks.

Within a week, clothes had been delivered to them from their quarters in Sicily, and everyone but Jens and Sergeant Cruise, who was diagnosed with pneumonia, was released to return to the squadron in Sicily.

09 January 1944, Sunday—1730: OSS Headquarters, Bari

Captain Lloyd Smith had just completed his report of the evacuation mission and was standing in front of a mirror in a washroom adjacent to his office, shaving. He heard the office door open and close and footsteps approaching, and turned to see a man extending his hand. Surprised, he recognized General William "Wild Bill" Donovan, director of the Office of Strategic Services. Smith took his hand and shook it.

"I wanted to congratulate you on the success of your mission," General Donovan said. "President Roosevelt has followed the situation daily and will be most pleased to learn of the group's safe return." He paused. "That is, all but the three nurses who are still in Albania."

"Yes, sir," Smith said. He wiped the shaving cream from the right side of his face with the corner of the towel draped around his neck. "Lieutenant Duffy, SOE, and others I've spoken with, believe that the women are in hiding in Berat."

"Yes, that's the intelligence I've received too," General Donovan said. He seated himself on the edge of Smith's desk. "Well, you're in for a furlough, Captain. Where would you like to go? Pick something good, because when you get back in a week or two, you'll be going back to Albania for the three nurses left behind."

Smith wasn't at all surprised, but he was delighted to be offered his choice of places for furlough.

"If it's all right with you, General, I'd like to go to Cairo. I've heard some of the men I went through training with are there, waiting for their next assignments."

"Fine," Donovan said. "Be at the airfield in three hours and a plane will take you directly to Cairo." He stood and shook hands with Smith again. "I'll be back in Washington in a month or two, and I'll personally tell President Roosevelt about your success. By that time, I should be able to include the success of your second mission to Albania."

"Yes, sir," Smith replied. "I'll get on it as soon as I return from Cairo."

09 January 1944, Sunday—1900: The Twenty-sixth General Hospital

Jens was pleasantly surprised to receive a visit from a freshly shaven and bathed Captain Lloyd Smith.

"Well, don't you look nice!" Jens said as he walked to the side of her bed. "I hardly recognized you without the dirt and lice—and your beard."

Smith smiled. "I can certainly say the same about you. How are you feeling?"

"Good, and getting better by the minute," Jens said. "I do have one little problem with a boil on my leg, but after they do an incision and drainage on it tomorrow, it should clear up in no time."

"With everything you've been through, I'm sure a boil is just a minor inconvenience," Smith said. He patted her arm. "I'll be leaving for a two weeks' furlough in a couple of hours, and I thought you might like to know that I already have my next assignment."

Their eyes met and without a specific word on the matter, Jens knew Smith would be returning to Albania to bring the other three nurses back to Allied territory.

"Thank you seems so inadequate," Jens said. "If it weren't for you and Gary, we might all be sitting in a German POW camp, right now." She squeezed Smith's hand. "Good luck on your next mission. I'll be waiting for word of its success."

Report of Lieutenant Gavin B. Duffy, SOE

09 January 1944
So the evacuation was completed. For the party in general,

they behaved splendidly, especially the nurses whose courage and faith were a tonic to the people escorting them on what might have been quite a disastrous journey. High tribute should be paid to Capt. SMITH who did magnificent work in the latter part of the journey. Tribute should also be paid to the people of the villages through which we passed, most of whom were extremely hospitable, even when a reprisal by the Germans would be the price to be paid.

14 Smith to the Rescue

Report of Major Lloyd G. Smith, OSS

Orders were received from the Commanding Officer, SBS on January 30, 1944 to proceed with the evacuation of the three American nurses of an air corps medical unit who were reported to be in the vicinity of BERAT.

Due to naval operations the American ship YANKEE was unable to leave its port at BRINDISI until 1000 hours February 2, 1944. It arrived at the base at SEAVIEW at 2300 hours of the same day.

At SEAVIEW I was met by Major Kendall (Dale McAdoo, SI). He informed me that several individuals who were quite prominent BALLISTS had promised to bring the nurses to the base. He suggested that I wait a few days at the base rather than set out for BERAT immediately. He said that if the nurses came with the men who had promised to bring them they would be at the base within the next ten days.

On or about 12 February 1944 the local representative of BALLI KOMBETAR began to worry a great deal over the safety of the two bases, SEAVIEW and SEA ELEPHANT. They were certain the Germans knew of our location and they thought it would be a matter of only a few days before we were attacked. I made a reconnaisance to the north of Seaview looking for possible bases and emergency hide-outs. On this recce Germans were spotted living in a house on a high point approximately two hundred meters north of Orso Bay.

Guards, (shepherds) were posted and instructed to inform us should the Germans decide to move south toward our bases. While I was away on this reconnaisance SKENDER MUCHO one of the prominent Ballists of VALONA visited GRAMMA BAY (Sea Elephant). Mucho had been unable to fulfill his promise to Major Kendall. He had promised to bring the nurses to the base. Because of my absence on reconnaissance I was unable to talk with Mucho on the occasion of his visit.

The situation was rather critical at this time because we were expecting the Germans any day and I did not care to risk leaving the base, pick up the nurses and return to find it in German hands.

On 24 February 1944, HODO METO, an English speaking local Ballist whom I had met on my first assignment in Albania came to Gramma Bay. His services were commandeered immediately for help in evacuating the nurses.

I had talked with Marine Corps Gy. Sergeant Nick Cooky (SI) and we agreed that when we received word that the Germans were coming he would hide his battery and we would go together taking his W/T set with him. In this way we would still have communications to arrange for bringing a ship to some safe place along the southern cost [coast] for evacuation.

With the help of Hodo Meto, letters were written to MITDHAT FRASHERI and CADRE CAKRON. They were informed of my specific assignment and that several members of their organization had promised to bring the nurses to the base and had done nothing; that the United States Army knew the nurses were with them and under their care and if they were not evacuated within a certain lenght [length] of time I would be asked for reasons and would be obliged to state that my failure was due to a lack of cooperation on the part of Balli Kombetar. Hodo was to send the letters with his cousin who he assured me is very reliable and exactly the man for the assignment. This cousin was provided with money to secure credentials and to purchase civilian cloths [clothes] for the nurses to make the trip from Berat by automobile should they decide to get out of uniform. In my letter to the nurses, I told them the decision as to whether or not they wished to change to civilian clothes and make the trip by car or have me come up and bring them down by foot was entirely theirs.

Hodo was very much opposed to the idea of my going to Berat on foot and bringing the nurses down to the base since he knew that I would insist on his accompanying me and that we would have to pass through some Partisan-held territory. He also could not understand why the nurses should have any decision in the matter. He remarked, "We always tell our women what to do."

This same night at 2000 hrs. we received word that the Germans, four of them were coming and were one hour north of Seaview. Major Quayle, senior BLO at the base ordered Gramma Bay to be evacuated and we moved East two hours to await further developments.

On the morning of 25 February 1944 Sgt. Cooky with his radio equipment joined me at our hiding place in accordance with our previous plan. He informed me that he had hidden a battery before leaving Seaview.

At 1000 hours on the 26th, four Germans moved into Gramma Bay. Other Germans were reported to be coming up from the south. Major Quayle divided the personnel into three groups and instructed them to reunite on the other side of the mountain in the village of DUKATI. Hodo wanted to know if we should proceed with our plans for the evacuation of the nurses. After assuring him that we still could evacuate the nurses successfully in spite of the Germans, he started for the village of Dukati to send his cousin to Berat with the messages.

Sgt. Cooky and I travelled up the mountain to the snowline. He carried his W/T equipment and I carried the packs of both. We waited in a gulley at the snowline until dusk and then started towards the top. After travelling for four hours in knee-deep snow and walking against a wing [wind] that was knocking us off our feet every few yards, we decided to come back down the mountain a few hundred yards and find shelter. At this time we came into a hard rain. That night we bundled together under a rock ledge with our two blankets. The next morning I had the feeling that I had not slept at all, however Sgt. Cooky insisted that I was both snoring and shivering, not just shivering. We were still above the snowline.

The next morning, 27 February 1944, we spotted six Germans who were coming south from Orso Bay. At almost exactly the same time we were spotted by them. We tricked them into believing that we were going down the mountain and then continued on our way over the top. Sgt. Cooky and I between us had two K-rations which we made last for three days. Everyone reached Dukati within the next two days.

About ten days later we discovered that the Germans had overlooked our base at Seaview. Major Quayle then decided that Seaview would be used only to receive sorties and that nor [no] personnel would make extended stops there. Since the Germans were fully aware of the fact that we were in that area this was a very wise decision.

Since I had received no word about the nurses by 10 March 1944 another messenger was sent to Berat. Hodo kept assuring me all the while that his cousin would return shortly with the nurses. He went so far as to state, "If my cousin does not return within ten days, you can shoot me. I'll bet my life on him."

On March 14, 1944 I received a message from Cairo telling me, "If nurses can be successfully evacuated in next thirty days continue, if not, return to Bari without further instructions." This message worried Hodo greatly. It was then decided that if the nurses had not arrived by the 21st or if we had no word from them he and I would start on foot to Berat. Although he was greatly worried he continued to express absolute confidence in his cousin.

Later, Jens learned the rest of the story.

When Wilma Lytle, Ann Maness, and Helen Porter were awakened by gunfire in Berat on the morning of November 15, 1943, they didn't rush to the street as their companions did; instead, they listened to their hosts, who urged them to go with the family to a hiding place in their basement. As soon as the bombing stopped, the streets were filled with German tanks and soldiers, and the girls realized then that they could not attempt to escape. Their hosts assured them that they could keep them safe.

German soldiers came that very day to search the house. They spoke to the nurses, who identified themselves as Americans, but the two German soldiers, for whatever reason, did not report them. Their host and his family, some of whom spoke English, were members of the Ballista and had many influential friends within the party, including a commandant who was very helpful. The family dug a hole through the basement wall between their house and the house next door, the home of the host's cousin. When word was passed that the three American women had gone, the three were able to hide in the cousin's house whenever necessary.

The three nurses did not lack for food or comfort during their confinement, and with the help of an Albanian-English dictionary they could communicate. Time passed slowly, however, and by February they began to fear that not enough effort was being made by the Albanians for their evacuation. In desperation they told their host that they thought they should try to get to the coast on their own. The family dissuaded them, and once again the commandant came to reassure them of their safety for as long as was necessary.

15 March 1944:
Berat

Two English-speaking Albanians came to the house to tell them of a plan for their escape. The women were given Albanian names, passes with their pictures, and clothing of Albanian style, including large black scarves to cover their heads and part of their faces.

18 March 1944

The Albanian in charge of the plan came to the house, and he and the three nurses slipped through the basement exit and out the cousin's back door into a waiting car. The car was followed by a truckload of Albanian soldiers. When they were stopped by German patrols, the driver showed a letter giving them permission for the trip, ostensibly to transport the soldiers to an area to fight partisans. In this way they were able to travel by car until they were well out of Berat. Then the car and truck turned back, and the nurses and one Albanian guide continued their journey on foot, walking along dirt roads and trails. They spent the night in a shepherd's hut and resumed their trek the next day. In the late afternoon they reached a house where two British soldier were waiting. The soldiers ran on ahead to tell the American officer, Major Lloyd G. Smith, OSS, that the women had arrived in the area and would wait for him at a deserted house.

Report of Major Lloyd G. Smith, OSS

19 March 1944 [Hideout, near southwestern Albanian coast]
    On the 19th, I was awakened at 0700 hours by a very excited English corporal. He was standing in the hut where I was sleeping. His suspenders were dangling down the sides of his trousers and his gun belt was doing the work his suspenders should have been doing. Seeing him in such a state of excitement and figuring that he was warning me of the approaching Germans I reached for my gun belt and panic pack. His first coherent words of "the nurses have arrived" brought me to my feet faster than any Germans could have. Hodo's first words were, "See, God-damit, Major, I told you my cousin would bring them." I met the nurses on the trail and brought them to the shepherd's hut where I was staying.
    Hodo's cousin had gone to Berat and had supervised the carrying out of my plans of having credentials and clothing made for the nurses to come down by automobile. He did a beautiful piece of work and deserves all credit for their successful evacuation. The fact that credentials had to be secured in TIRANA [Tiranë], the capital, delayed the nurses in getting started. Suleyman Mecho who speaks very fluent

English accompanied the party from Berat and acted as their interpreter.

The nurses were in the best possible physical condition when they arrived and spoke very highly of the care they had received from the Balli Kombetar.

Mecho expressed a great desire to have American officers come in to work with the Balli Kombetar to prepare them for action against the Germans when they move out of Albania.

Through Hodo's good connection in Dukati, two liters of gasoline were purchased in order that Corporal Crane could charge a battery and get on the air long enough to send a message to SBS for me.——Sgt. Cooky had gone back to Seaview to help receive a sortie.

On the evening of the 19th, under [cover] of darkness, the nurses were taken down the Valona-Dukati Road to the house of Xhelil Chela. We arrived at this house at 2030 hours.

At 0230 hours on 20 March 1944 we left the house and started up the mountain. By day break we were high enough on the mountain to be out of sight of any Germans who might be passing on the Valona-Dukati Road. The dise [face] of the mountain as we climbed was covered with snow from five hundred meters up to the top. We reached the top at 1100 hours. Reached Seaview at 1415 hours. The nurses were given the most comfortable cave to recuperate from their very tiring hike.

At 2330 hours 21 March 1944, we left the coast of Albania in an Italian MTB. The nurses were very seasick. We arrived at OTRANTO at 0130 hours on March 22, 1944 were [where] we had tea aboard a Yugoslav yacht and rested until morning. Nurses were then taken to HQ SBS in an ambulance, after which they were taken to the 26th General Hospital.
Signed: Lloyd Smith, Major, AUS.

And so the last of the thirty stranded Americans returned, and the Albanian escape was complete.

Epilogue

On 21 January 1944 Lieutenant Agnes Jensen was released from the hospital and returned to her squadron in Sicily. In accordance with military policy that anyone who had crash-landed in and escaped from enemy territory could not remain in the same theater of war, orders were waiting for her, and on 23 January she began the first leg of her journey back to the United States.

When Jens arrived at her parents' farm, she learned that the military had contacted her parents on 26 November 1943 and informed them that she was missing in enemy territory. One week later, on Jens's birthday, her parents received a second telegram informing them that their daughter was alive, in Allied hands, and that they should hear from her soon. Today, Jens confesses with a smile that she never told her parents that she had volunteered as a flight nurse.

After three weeks at home on leave and ten days at a relocation center in Atlantic City, she returned to duty at Bowman Field, Kentucky, as an instructor in the flight nurse training program. Part of her regular assignment was to accompany trainees on their first flights to New York, Presque Isle, Miami, and San Francisco, where they picked up patients returning from all battle fronts.

Shortly after being assigned to Bowman Field Jens got orders to tour the United States on a war bond drive—and on that tour she experienced her second crash-landing when their C-47 had trouble over Spirit Lake, Iowa, and the pilot had to feather one of his two engines. The pilot decided to set down on a nearby civilian field that had been used by crop dusters and other small planes. Jens looked out of the window as the aircraft turned to line up with the runway.

At least the people on the ground will speak English, she thought as she registered the too-short field and the fact that they were flying on only one engine. The plane hit the runway squarely and began to roll at a pretty good speed. Jens and her companions were thrown forward as the pilot applied the brakes. They were out of runway before they were out of steam. The C-47 lurched as its wheels left concrete for dirt and came to rest with its nose firmly against a large tree.

As they deplaned, Jens said to the pilot, "This is my second crash-landing in less than a year."

The pilot said, "Any landing you can walk away from is a *good* landing!"

In the early summer of 1945 Jens unexpectedly met Thrasher at an army airfield. After they got caught up on each other's doings, she asked him whether he had heard anything about Duffy. Unfortunately Thrasher told her Duffy had been killed while parachuting into Berlin in 1944.

In late July 1945 Jens visited Cleveland and telephoned Kostig Steffa's brother. The Steffas were happy to hear from her. In less than an hour, George, Telemak and their wives met Jens at her hotel and talked over a long lunch.

Not until 1993 did Jens learn that contrary to what Thrasher had told her in 1945, Gavin Duffy had not died in Berlin. He had remained in the British army following the war and had retired as the director of an army recruiting center, with the rank of major. He died in 1990, at the age of seventy. Jens was saddened to realize that when she was in England in 1976 she could have sought out Duffy, had she not believed that he was dead.

Jens married soon after World War II and traveled extensively with her husband, a government tax expert, and their two children.

Major Lloyd G. Smith retired from the army with the rank of Lieutenant Colonel. He and his wife became close friends of Jens and her husband. Until recently the two families lived within fifty miles of each other and visited and spoke frequently by telephone.

In 1995, accompanied by her son, Jon, and her daughter, Karen, Jens returned to Albania. At Steffa's home she talked for some time his widow. Steffa had been executed by the Communists in an Albanian prison near Berat in 1947. She also discovered that Steffa's oldest son, Alfredo, to whom she had given her flight wings, was ill and in the hospital. He died the following day, before Jens could visit him. When she inquired about Hassan, she was informed that he had died in 1988.

In 1996, Lloyd G. Smith traveled to Albania as well. Shortly after he returned home the American Embassy in Albania forwarded him a letter from Quani Sigeca, who, as a young teenager, had been known to Jens's group as "Johnny" and had acted as a guide to the Americans for several days following the bombing and strafing of Berat.

In 1997, when her son and grandchildren were visiting, Jens listened as Jon read a bedtime story to Christopher, nine years old, and Jonathan, eight. He read the boys the manuscript for this book, telling of their grandmother's crash landing in and escape from Albania, leaving their image of Grandma forever changed. On a visit to the Smithsonian Air and Space Museum the following day, in the midst of a large crowd, Jonathan pointed at the C-47 suspended from the ceiling. Heads turned as the clear and resonant voice of an eight-year-old asked, "Is that Grandma's plane she crashed in Albania with— or is it her plane that crashed with its nose against a tree?"

Glossary

a/c: aircraft

Adj: Adjutant

AFHQ: Air Force Headquarters

armd: armored

APO: Army Post Office

AUS: Army of the United States

Ballist: An Albanian pro-Nazi militaristic group

BLO: British Liaison Officer

British mission: a designation for any location where one or more British intelligence operatives were "in residence"; the British mission moved from place to place as enemy movements necessitated.

bullybeef: canned or pickled beef

CG: Commanding General

challenge: a military term referring to a sentry's call, requiring one to halt and give the countersign

CMA: Chief Military Authority

CQ: Charge of Quarters

DDD: Duffy's wireless coded signature

EAOBH: Northern Epirote National Liberation Organization, a local resistance group which was a branch of the Greek National Democratic League (EDES)

ETA: estimated time of arrival

GMT: Greenwich Mean Time

Gp: Group

grd: ground
G.S.: government service
GSC: General Service Command
HQ: headquarters
Incl: include or inclusive
in quin: five copies
leagur [leaguer]: any military camp
LNC: Liberation National Committee: Albanian pro-Communist partisan group
M. 2912, etc.: reference to military map markings
MAES: Medical Air Evacuation Squadron
M.I.: Military Intelligence
military alphabet: e.g., Oboe Sugar Sugar = OSS; Uncle Sugar = U.S.
military time: examples, 0100 = 1:00 A.M..; 0200 = 2:00 A.M.; 1200 = 12:00 noon; 1300 = 1:00 P.M., etc.
MTs: military tanks
NATOUSA: North African Theater of Operations United States Army
OAF: Office of the Air Force, an army post office directional
OSS: U.S. Office of Strategic Services
PD: period
PU: pick up
QRK, QRZ: wireless radio frequencies
"railroad tracks": military slang for Army captain's insignia
rochi: an alcoholic drink of the Balkans region, frequently brewed at home
rpt: repeat
SAS: Special Air Services
SBS: Special Bari Section (OSS Balkan Operations)
SHTABIT: local military commandant
sitrep: situation report
sked: scheduled

SOE: Special Operations Executive, a branch of British intelligence working mainly behind enemy lines.

SOP: standard operating procedure

Sq: Squadron

T3: technical sergeant (T/Sgt.), level 3, an army enlisted rating

TC: Transportation Corps

unmarked planes: Unlike hospital trains and ships that were marked with red crosses and used only for transporting casualties, military aircraft that transported flight nurses, medics, and wounded were also used to transport troops and equipment and therefore were not marked with red crosses.

VE: Victory in Europe

worry beads: Muslim beads numbering thirty-three or multiples thereof, used to keep count while reciting a zikr or verse

W/T: wireless transmitter

Bibliography

Boyle, Harold V. "Nurses Met Blizzard, Bombs, and Civil War on Albania Trek." *Baltimore Sun*, 16 February 1944.

Duffy, 1st Lt. Gavin B., British Mission, Albania. "A Report on Evacuation of the American Party from Albania, 1943." January 1944, author's archives.

"German Antiguerrilla Operations in the Balkans (1941-1944)." CMH Publication 104-18, National Archives, Washington, D.C.

"How Nurses Dodged Nazis." *New York Sun*, 16 February 1944.

HQ, NATOUSA. "Memorandum to Commanding General, Army Air Forces, Washington, DC." 29 November 1943. National Archives, Washington, D.C., RG112.32.

"The Incredible Journey." *Daily Post* (Liverpool, England), 28 February 1995.

Infield, Glenn B. *Disaster at Bari*. New York: Bantam Books, 1988.

Kennly, 1st Lt. William H., XII Troop Carrier Command, APO 760. "Memorandum to Commanding General, 12th Air Force, APO 650." 19 November 1943. National Archives, Washington, D.C., RG112.32.

Landsberg, Dr. H. "No. 193, The Strategic Aspects of Balkan Climate." Institute of Meteorology, University of Chicago, for the Weather Research Center. September 1942. National Archives, Washington, D.C.

Marmullaku, Ramadan. *Albania and the Albanians*. London: Archon Books, 1975.

Porter, Amy. "Balkan Escape." *Collier's*, 1 April 1944.

"Rescued from Albania, American Nurses Adventure." *Times* (London), 16 February 1944.

Ruches, Pyrrhus. *Albania's Captives*. Chicago: Argonaut, 1965.

Skendk, Stavro, ed. *Albania*. New York: Praeger, 1956.

Smith, Lloyd G., (Capt.). "Report on Mission of Evacuation, American Rescue Party: Period November 30, 1943 to January 9, 1944." Courtesy of Lloyd G. Smith, Lt. Col., AUS (Ret.).

———, (Maj.). "Evacuation of Three American Nurses from Albania: 29 March 1944." Courtesy of Lloyd G. Smith, Lt. Col., AUS (Ret.).

———, (Lt. Col., AUS [Ret.]). Interviews by authors, October 1996–April 1997.

"Stanwood Nurse Tells of Experience in Enemy Land." *Big Rapids (Mich.) Pioneer,* 25 February 1944.

Stinson, Col. David, GSC, Chief of Staff. "Memorandum to Major General Smith, AFHQ." 29 November 1943. National Archives, Washington, D.C.

Sixty-first Troop Carrier Squadron, Army Air Forces, Office of the Operations Officer. "Missing Aircraft Memorandum." 13 November 1943. National Archives, Washington, D.C.

314th Troop Carrier Group, Army Air Force, Office of Group Commander. "Missing Air Crew Report." 15 November 1943. National Archives, Washington, D.C.

Winnifrith, Tom, ed. *Perspectives on Albania.* London: Macmillan, 1992.

Yarbrough, T.E. Letter to author, 17 November 1994.